"It is one thing to intellectually understand what faith looks like during trials; and altogether something else to experience how faith feels and grows during the trial itself. In Diane McGovern's book, *Our Ever-Present Help*, she skillfully takes the reader through the raw and winding emotions that her own family experienced as their daughter teetered between life and death. You will follow the ups and downs of their often-circuitous spiritual journey.

I highly recommend this book as it will not only spur you on in your own faith, it will comfort, encourage, and prepare you to experience God-sized help in your own life.

> Judy Gerry, Ancient Paths Ministries and author of *Facing Adversity*, a Bible study"

Our Ever-Present Help

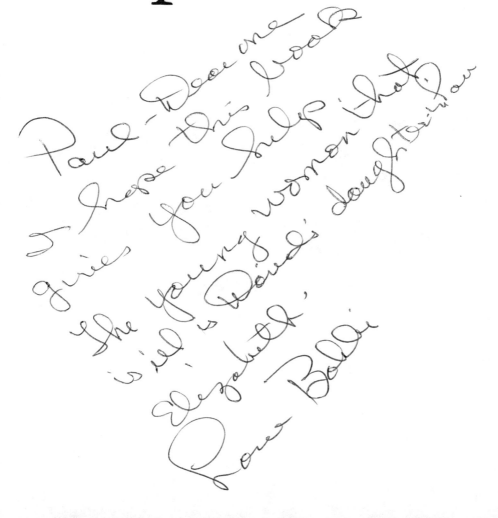

Paul — Dear one
I hope this book
gives you help that
the young women that
wed — David's daughter-in-law
Elizabeth,
Love, Billi

Our Ever-Present Help

A Family's Journey Through a Life-Threatening Lung Disease

Diane McGovern

WestBow Press
A DIVISION OF THOMAS NELSON

Copyright © 2012 Diane McGovern

All rights reserved. No part of this book may be used or reproduced by any means—graphic, electronic, or mechanical, including photocopying, recording, taping or by any information storage retrieval system without the written permission of the publisher, except in the case of brief quotations embodied in critical articles and reviews.

Scripture taken from the HOLY BIBLE, NEW INTERNATIONAL VERSION®. Copyright © 1973, 1978, 1984 by International Bible Society. Used by permission of Zondervan. All rights reserved.

Scripture quotations taken from the New American Standard Bible®, Copyright © 1960, 1962, 1963, 1968, 1971, 1972, 1973, 1975, 1977, 1995 by THE LOCKMAN FOUNDATION. Used by permission. (www.Lockman.org)

Scripture taken from the Amplified Bible, Copyright © 1954, 1958, 1962, 1964, 1965, 1987 by The Lockman Foundation. Used by permission.

WestBow Press books may be ordered through booksellers or by contacting:
WestBow Press
A Division of Thomas Nelson
1663 Liberty Drive
Bloomington, IN 47403
www.westbowpress.com
1-(866) 928-1240

Because of the dynamic nature of the Internet, any web addresses or links contained in this book may have changed since publication and may no longer be valid. The views expressed in this work are solely those of the author and do not necessarily reflect the views of the publisher, and the publisher hereby disclaims any responsibility for them.

Any people depicted in stock imagery provided by Thinkstock are models, and such images are being used for illustrative purposes only.

Certain stock imagery © Thinkstock.

ISBN: 978-1-4497-4754-1 (sc)
ISBN: 978-1-4497-4755-8 (hc)
ISBN: 978-1-4497-4753-4 (e)

Library of Congress Control Number: 2012906590

Printed in the United States of America
WestBow Press rev. date: 5/24/2012

For my husband, Matt—thank you for standing by me and listening tirelessly through my writing journey. Together we learned that a project like this is no small task.

As a person who starts more projects than I finish, I could see many opportunities along the way to give up. Plowing through many edits made me feel that actually finishing the book was a novel idea. But you picked me up repeatedly and encouraged me to press on toward completion.

"Just finish it!" you pleaded. "You've already worked on this for such a long time. Just get it done!"

I needed that.

You've also been willing to let me share personally about our marriage in the book, which was not part of my original plan. Exposing weaknesses and boasting in them so Christ's power may be seen is easier said than done. Thank you for your courage to accompany me there. I'm grateful the Lord taught us He's never finished working in our lives, no matter how old we are.

I'm so thankful for the privilege to continue our adventure in Christ—together. I'm still yours—Diane.

"In times like these you need a savior
In times like these you need an anchor
Be very sure, be very sure
Your anchor holds and grips the Solid Rock!
This Rock is Jesus, Yes, He's the One
This Rock is Jesus, the only One!"[1]

Ruth Caye Jones

---

[1] "In Times Like These", words and music by Ruth Caye Jones ©1944 New Spring Publishing (ASCAP). All Rights Reserved. Used By Permission.

Contents

Acknowledgements		xi
Introduction	Whatever It Takes	xiii
Chapter 1	Losing Control	1
Chapter 2	Something Drastic	13
Chapter 3	God's Place of Refuge	25
Chapter 4	God At Work	39
Chapter 5	Surrender	51
Chapter 6	Spiritual Roller Coaster	61
Chapter 7	Perfect, Faithful Provision	70
Chapter 8	"How Long, O Lord?" (Psalm 13:1a)	82
Chapter 9	A Firm Foundation	96
Chapter 10	"I Love Jesus—He Is My Strength"	108
Chapter 11	The Lord Finally Had Me Where He Wanted Me	123
Chapter 12	Dance	136
Chapter 13	From Bad to Worse	146
Chapter 14	Burden Bearers	156
Chapter 15	The Shepherd's Voice	169
Chapter 16	Longsuffering	182
Chapter 17	Plans for a Hope and a Future	195
Chapter 18	Testify	210
Epilogue		223
Resources		229

Acknowledgements

God used many dedicated medical professionals including excellent teams of doctors, nurses, respiratory therapists, and physical therapists; 27 fervently praying churches; countless prayer chains, Bible studies, prayer groups; and even strangers who prayed. We are so grateful for all of your help on our daughter's behalf.

Other ministries and groups that prayed include:
Advent Ministries, Alabaster, Azusa Pacific University, Bellflower Friendship Manor, Bible Study Fellowship-Ventura, CA, Biola University-Admissions Dept./Hart Hall-HUOD (Elizabeth's dorm)/Psychology Dept./Security Dept./Telecounselors/Uganda Missions Team-Summer 2004, Body Builders, Caleb Community, Calvary Chapel Bible College, Camarillo Christian Women's Club, Cornerstone Christian School, Christian Mission School-Uganda, Eastside Christian School, Healthy Habits, Hume Lake Couples Retreat, Joshua Wilderness Training-Hume Lake, Keenagers Sunday School Class, San Gabriel Christian School, Sojourners Sunday School Class, The Palms-La Mirada, CA, Trinity Broadcasting-700 Club, and Whittier Christian School.

And thank you from our family to each of these precious, supportive individuals:

Dave Anderson, Luc Alexander, Sam Alexander, Jennifer Alvarez (Moyer), Emily Balyut (Torres), Brian, Shireen, Spring and Jade Batstone, Charlie

Begg, Dave Blosat, Ron and Jane Boyer, Elyse, Jimmy and Sissy Burks, Jack and Elsie Burks, Anne Burson, Ralph Butler, Matt Cain, Karen Carlisle, Carol Chrysong, Jeri Chrysong, Jerry and Rose Mary Chrysong, Dave Clelland, Annette Close, Doug Coe, Clyde Cook, Tracy Corbett, Dan and Shirley Coulter, Auston Cronk, Beth Cronk (Moyer), John and Heather Curtis, Marty Daly, Cheryl Daniels, Becky Dean (Tittel), Hope DeMoss, Chrysti Dena, Michelle Devine, Suzanne Dykstra, Cindy Ehde, Sandi Edwards, Kevin Erickson, Abbey Ervin, Heidi Fiske (Youngdale), Mike Ford, Judy Fox, Renee Gauthier, Judy Gerry, Cheryl and Heather Gillaspy, Brad Gist, Brian and Cathe Gordon, Linda Graveline, Caitlyn Gregorich, John Gregorich, Ruth Gunderson, Tracy Hackney, Michael and Terry Harriton, Barbara Hicks, Kenneth and Marion Holladay and family, Wayne Hopkins, Nancy Howison, George and Myrna Huisken, Michael Joe, Mary Kays, Kenny Kibble, Pam Kilduff, Elizabeth Kliner, Katherine Kniss, Delores Kootz, John Krutsinger, Nancy Kuthy, Tim Larson, Sal and Patsy Lopez, Ryan Lowe, Susan Ludes, Marie Milla, Mary March, Evonne Marshall, Joy Matthews, Sarah McClaran, Denise McCormick, Darlene McGovern, Ed McGovern, Sister Shirley McGovern, Steven and Caroline Mercer, Dave Miller, Cee Cee Mills, Brett Mitchell, Bob and June Morris, Joel and Rosemary Morris, Rachel Morris, Jim and Gayle Moyer, Tammy, Eleanor, and Anna Mudica, Emily Neimeyer, Christa Norby, Scott Packham, Nick Padron, Pat Papenhausen, Kenneth Parker, Megan Parker (Moyer), Dave Patrick, Dorothy Pettigrew, Paul and Donna Phillipps and family, Bruce and Billie Pryor, Pat Rees, Ralph Rittenhouse, Nancy Rodriguez, Tami Rutledge, Bob and Darlene Sheets, Frank and Nancy Sheets, Cari Schnars, Haiyan J. Schopke, Barbara Smith, Brian Smith, Marilyn Smith, Terry and Linda Sneed, Howard Speaks, Mike and Debbie Stanton, Joy Strawbridge, Kevin Tasker, Tony Terry, Karen Thompson, Karen Tittel, Carolyn Trotter, Cheryl West (Urke), Jeff Urke, Darlene Vanlandingham, Barbara Velji, Candace Webb, Betty Welch, Fred and Betty Wilkin, and Matt Williams.

INTRODUCTION

Whatever It Takes

I COULDN'T GET MY MIND off of new teaching I'd just heard at Bible study on Romans 8:28—

> "And we know that God causes all things to work together for good to those who love God, to those who are called according to His purpose" (NASB).

The teacher had beautifully unfolded the meaning. ALL things, even the worst suffering, can be used by God to conform us to the image of His Son, Jesus. He alone has the power to use negative effects to generate new, positive outcomes.

As I kept thinking, my deepest, secret agony came to mind.

"Lord, what about the spiritual disharmony in my marriage?" I asked Him. "Why do we fight so much about walking in faith?"

My husband, Matt, and I were both believers. Even so, sharing truth and encouraging each other rarely happened. We'd agreed early on to live on one income while I stayed home to raise our family. Trusting God with tight finances began creating great animosity between us. From my perspective, Matt grew more and more fearful and angry through the years.

"I can't respect his leadership because he's telling me not to trust You, Lord," I prayed. "You've proven Yourself faithful. How can You make this work for good?"

"Often a work of God comes with two edges, great joy and great pain,"[2] said Philip Yancey in his book *The Jesus I Never Knew*.

He discusses the difficulties of Mary's unplanned parenthood. She was willing to do anything God wanted, no matter what it would cost her personally. In her obedience, we see her embrace both great joy and great pain.

By the time our children were teenagers, still nothing "good" had worked out. In Matt's heart, fear and anger were dominant. I felt a little like Paul when he said:

"I have great sorrow and unceasing anguish in my heart" (Romans 9:2).

Paul wished his own loss of Christ if it would benefit his people. I wasn't ready to go that far, but I wondered what it would take to create spiritual harmony in our 20-year-old marriage.

"A rebuilt car engine will cost $1,700.00," a mechanic told Matt one day. When I heard the bad news, my body tensed up. I was sure that huge bill would push him way over the edge. When I suggested we pray about it, I knew how he'd react.

"We can't come up with that much money!" said Matt, highly agitated.

"I'm not getting into this argument again!" I said as I left the room.

I began the next morning in tears. When I got up, the dresser mirror reflected dreary, lifeless eyes from a hopeless face. I longed for change more than ever.

Just then, the Holy Spirit broke through, whispering a daring idea into my heart.

Consider this prayer: "Do whatever it takes for my husband to grow spiritually again." Are you willing to pray like that?

Surprised at God's bold message, I had to stop and think.

"Lord! You've never asked me to pray such an extreme prayer before. Are You asking my permission to do something drastic?"

---

[2] Philip Yancey, <u>The Jesus I Never Knew</u>, #32, © 1995. Reprinted by permission. Thomas Nelson Inc., Nashville, Tennessee. All rights reserved.

My brain kept trying to take in God's holy suggestion. It sounded risky.

"What could 'whatever it takes' mean?" I thought. "Maybe He'll allow me to get cancer or even die. Hmmm, is it worth it to me to suffer so a spiritual change of heart can take place in someone else? How valuable is just one vibrant spiritual life to God?"

Diane, you wanted Me to work. Now let Me do something, the Lord said.

Ready to surrender to God's request, I got down on my knees to pray.

"Lord, do whatever it takes for my husband to grow spiritually again. I want headway to occur, even if it means I'll suffer. I really mean this."

I didn't see anything happen right away. From time to time, I repeated my prayer, reminding God I was serious about it. But in the busyness of life, I'd halfway forgotten about it. Our struggle intensified. Years passed.

However, God didn't forget my prayer. In His wisdom, He knew each member of my family needed to grow in faith. He was about to take our 22-year-old daughter, Elizabeth, and the rest of our family on a journey that would profoundly affect us all.

In the spring of 2004, He began implementing His drastic plan.

CHAPTER ONE

Losing Control

"I can't breathe very well," gasped Elizabeth from the floor of our bedroom. No one heard her when she'd called for help from the living room sometime after midnight. Afraid she'd pass out if she tried to walk, she used all her strength to crawl down the hall and burst into our room to wake us up.

Matt and I began stirring. "What's going on, Elizabeth?" Matt asked, still a little groggy from sleep.

"I think she said she can't breathe too well," I said. "Yesterday the doctor diagnosed her with a kidney infection, but I don't think that should affect her lungs."

Matt quickly got down on the floor to listen to Elizabeth's breathing.

"Does it sound any different to you?" I asked.

"I don't hear anything unusual," he said. Then he helped Elizabeth back to her bed so she could lie down.

Matt returned to our bedroom. On the edge of feeling frantic, we continued our fast discussion. "Didn't the doctor put her on an antibiotic?" he asked.

"Yes, he did," I said. "Do you think taking her to the hospital right now would be overreacting?"

Then I thought about Elizabeth's extremely healthy history. She hardly ever got sick and she was rarely one to complain. The fact that she didn't feel she could wait until morning meant something. I went to Elizabeth's room to check on her again. The fear registering in her eyes convinced me to get moving.

"Matt, I think I should rush her to the Emergency Room now," I said as I threw on some clothes. He agreed. I remembered she'd just changed insurance coverage. I knew we'd need to find her insurance card. Matt got on that. Then he called a doctor for approval before we left for the hospital. We decided he would stay home with our youngest daughter, Sarah, who remained asleep, completely unaware of our midnight emergency.

I helped Elizabeth into the car and drove her to St. John's Pleasant Valley Hospital in Camarillo, California—a five-minute drive from our home.

Thoughts raced through my mind as I drove. "She has to keep breathing! Breathing trouble is a big deal. I'm scared for Elizabeth."

Once we arrived, I walked her to the hospital side entrance. It was locked. "You're not thinking, Diane. Go to the emergency entrance," I told myself. That entrance was twenty yards away, but it was open. I ran back to where I'd left Elizabeth. She was lying flat on the ground working very hard to breathe! I quickly helped her up from the cement walkway and into the emergency room check-in area.

A nurse began an initial examination in a little room. "Well, Elizabeth seems to be hooked up to this machine correctly," she said. "I wonder why her blood saturation level isn't registering."

As the nurse remained puzzled about what was wrong with her equipment, I wondered what was wrong with my daughter's lungs. Clearly, *they* weren't working properly!

After the doctor examined her, he ordered chest x-rays. When he returned, he looked concerned. He'd read the x-rays. "It's a good thing you brought her in because she's a very sick young woman," he said. "She has Influenza A and double pneumonia in her lower lungs." He explained that "double" meant both lungs.

"We'll be keeping her in the hospital," he said finally.

The process was begun to arrange a room for Elizabeth. I left her for a few minutes to call Matt. I nervously pressed "Home" on my cell phone.

"She's worse than I originally thought," he said after I told him how sick she was. We made new plans for the next morning, which was Sarah's 18th birthday.

At around four o'clock in the morning—hours after we'd arrived—Elizabeth was wheeled from the ER to an acute care isolated room on the second floor. I felt uneasy as I walked alongside her bed. My mind was troubled by thoughts I couldn't process.

"My daughter is so sick she needs to be hospitalized. This is unreal."

They situated her in her room. Before they let me go in, they explained an important requirement for an isolated room. Since Elizabeth was considered highly contagious because of the Influenza A, anyone going into her room had to put on a disposable mask, gown, and a pair of latex gloves, dispose of them on the way out, and then suit up all over again if they returned later. I put on my first set. Then I sat in a chair in the corner of her room.

Eventually, Elizabeth dozed a little. My mind went back to her childhood days. She was a beautiful child with the biggest brown eyes. She was a loving, gentle, unselfish, and helpful little girl. She was also smart and loved to read, run, and go camping on family vacations. I remembered her first Yosemite camping trip when she was 1 ½ years old. One morning, we gave her a bath on the campsite picnic table in our plastic dishwashing tub. While we washed her little body, sunbeams filtered through lofty pine trees down to the forest floor. A park ranger on horseback rode through the campground. He got a kick out of our little girl having a delightful bath. Later, when we rode a shuttle bus toward the trailhead of a hike, she was crazy about sucking on a nearby bus seat railing. Every part of camping was fun to her.

It was hard to reconcile the healthy, active person I'd always known her to be with this young woman in a hospital bed, struggling with each breath. "If only she was well," I thought longingly, "and we were leaving on a trip tonight instead of spending the night here!" I shut my tired eyes. I took time to exhale and pray.

"Thank you, Lord, for getting her to a place where she'll get help."

One week earlier…"I have too much to do this afternoon!" thought Elizabeth. "If I hurry, I can get to Rosemead to turn in my application for graduate school." Then I can run to the Uganda mission trip meeting. I'm glad I got my application to the Azusa Pacific University graduate school in the morning mail today along with my San Jose job application. There wouldn't have been time to get those done later."

Elizabeth, a psychology major in her senior year at Biola University in Southern California, had a schedule that was running her ragged. At that time, her studies were intense. She also felt there was never enough time to see John, her boyfriend and a fellow Biola student.

"I'm so excited to be graduating, but I don't think I can take anymore," Elizabeth said later as she rushed to change into her "server" pants and blouse to work the dinner shift at the nearby retirement residence. "I wish I didn't have to work this part time job—it demands hours I just don't have right now," she complained. "I'm so overwhelmed!"

After the dinner shift, Elizabeth returned to her dorm to start studying. That's when her body began aching all over. Her eyes burned and ached as well. She felt weak.

"I've got to lie down," she thought, making the tough climb into her dorm bed in the high bunk bed position. "But I still have a long list of things to finish by tomorrow," she cried. "How am I ever going to get everything done?"

Tears filled her burning eyes. They began streaming down her cheeks as she laid her head down. A large wet circle slowly formed on her pillow.

When her roommate returned later, she heard an achy moan from the direction of Elizabeth's bed.

"Are you okay, Elizabeth?" she asked.

"No," said Elizabeth. "I don't feel so good. I ache all over."

Her roommate asked if she could get her anything.

"I just need to sleep," said Elizabeth.

The next morning was the beginning of spring break. Elizabeth felt worse. "I'll be able to get over this when I'm home," she thought, as she began the one-and-a-half hour trip north of Biola. She forced herself to keep her eyes open so she'd stay alert enough to drive. The additional freeway traffic made the trip seem endless. "I really want to lie down in my bed," was her main thought. "I need my bed!"

Matt and I had looked forward to having her home over spring break. Once she arrived, we hugged her at the door. She greeted us in her usual loving way. Then she crashed into her bed. We'd never seen her so exhausted. We had no idea she felt so sick.

I was happy just having her near us again, sleeping under our roof. I realized how much I'd missed her. Matt and I were proud of the young woman she was becoming. It made me think of the woman she was named after. Although there were a few fine women named Elizabeth in my husband's family line, we named our first baby girl after the Elizabeth in the Bible, the wife of Zechariah and the late-in-life mother of John the Baptist.

I easily saw similarities in these two women named Elizabeth as our daughter became a young adult. Each lived an upright life in the sight of God. Each Elizabeth was a Spirit-filled woman who could see God working His plan out in the world. When He showed His favor to them personally, both women knew He was the One to praise.

I appreciated the ability Elizabeth and I had to share on a deep spiritual level before she even left for college. I recalled Elizabeth's faithful prayer support when she was a student leader in her church high school group. In her junior year, she and a few other students began meeting to pray before the regular Wednesday night youth ministry began. They prayed for students who were struggling with important relationships, school pressures, and faith issues. She lifted students up to God who resisted salvation. "I know they need the Lord. We'll just keep praying," she'd say.

Sometimes on Sunday mornings, she'd share a Bible verse that had spoken to her during the week from her quiet time. She'd write it out in the corner of the white board before high school worship began. As a volunteer youth worker, my own faith was encouraged one morning when I read one of her favorite verses repeatedly throughout the meeting.

"What is more, I consider everything a loss compared to the surpassing greatness of knowing Christ Jesus my Lord, for whose sake I have lost all things. I consider them rubbish, that I may gain Christ" (Philippians 3:8).

Back at the hospital, Matt and Sarah were putting on the protective gowns, gloves, and masks in the hall outside Elizabeth's room. Earlier that morning, Matt had gone into Sarah's bedroom with an unusual birthday greeting for her. Our family usually milks birthdays for all they're worth. We start the day by enthusiastically waking up the birthday girl to tell her "happy birthday" before she even gets out of bed. Then we gather in our living room to continue the celebration by giving presents. We usually plan a special outing chosen by the person with the birthday.

But that morning, Sarah was all warm and cozy when Matt knelt down beside her bed. "Sarah, wake up," he said. Although his face was serious, Sarah wasn't awake enough yet to notice.

As she slowly came to life, she remembered it was her birthday. Her face lit up with excitement. It was then that she noticed her father was alone with a worried expression on his face.

"Happy Birthday, Sarah. You're 18!" he said. Then he hesitated for a moment. "I kind of have some bad news. Your mom had to take Elizabeth to the hospital last night," he said.

Her dad gave her a short explanation of what had happened during the night. Still half awake, Sarah did her best to process everything. Then he suggested she get up and get ready so they could go to the hospital. He waited for her to move, to make sure she wouldn't go back to sleep.

Finally, she sat up. "Wait . . . what?" she asked.

"Your mom thought you'd want to open your presents with Elizabeth," said Matt. "Would it be okay if we take them to the hospital and have you open them there?" he asked.

"I guess that's okay," said Sarah." But as she got ready to go, Sarah felt disappointed.

"It's my eighteenth birthday! We have big plans," Sarah thought.

As Matt and Sarah walked into Elizabeth's room, Sarah stifled her irritation. She kindly greeted Elizabeth.

Even though very sick, Elizabeth was true to form. She didn't complain or demand attention. She dreaded the thought of ruining Sarah's birthday.

After a while, Sarah's heart softened. She knew she loved Elizabeth dearly. She started to understand that her big sister wasn't purposefully trying to ruin her birthday. Sarah hated to see her sister so sick.

After a brief visit, we gave Sarah her gifts. She smiled graciously as she opened them. Afterward, Sarah and Matt stayed with Elizabeth while I went home to get a few hours of sleep. Once I returned to the hospital, Matt and Sarah left. Sarah felt sad as they walked to the parking lot.

"I wanted Elizabeth to be part of my birthday celebration, but not like this," she said to her dad. "I want her home and for everything to be normal."

I suited up again in robe, mask, and gloves to spend time with Elizabeth. I sat down next to her bed. I studied her face. She looked pale and weak. Her tortured breathing combined with extreme nausea had etched a permanent painful expression on her face. Even so, she was trying to act normal. She carefully got out of bed to use the bathroom not long after I arrived. When she returned, she fell into bed, completely exhausted.

Her initial treatment included antibiotics, breathing treatments, and pain management. The need for strong medications and breathing treatments overwhelmed Elizabeth. Both her sisters had been diagnosed with asthma as little girls. They weren't strangers to breathing treatments. But Elizabeth didn't have asthma. This was all new to her. She's the type of person who never even takes aspirin for a headache.

All day, I longed to talk to Elizabeth's doctor, but he never came. When Matt returned to the hospital at 5:00 p.m., I went home. The doctor arrived just after I left. He introduced himself to Elizabeth and Matt, checked on her, and briefly discussed treatment plans.

When Matt returned home that evening, I realized the celebratory mood for Sarah's actual birthday had all but vanished since the morning. Her birthday ended with anxious parents at home and a sister in the hospital. We planned to have a party a few days later. I was hopeful that by then Elizabeth would be out of the hospital.

As I fell asleep at home that night, I had no idea Elizabeth was crying herself to sleep in the hospital. However, the next morning after I arrived, she informed me about an unfortunate experience with a respiratory therapist during a breathing treatment the night before. I'm sure he'd tried to motivate her by choosing to employ a firm manner while working with her. Instead it came off as harsh.

"Breathe deeper!" he'd barked.

Elizabeth was doing the absolute best she could. He saw no improvement.

"If you don't inhale the medicine more deeply, cough vigorously to loosen mucus, and then spit it out, you'll never get out of the hospital," he added disapprovingly.

True or not, his lack of compassion harassed Elizabeth's spirit.

After he left, Elizabeth felt miserable. "I want to be home," she cried in agony. She told me she wouldn't have wished her suffering on anyone—except maybe that respiratory therapist.

When Elizabeth finished her story, anger flared up inside me. "That guy was cruel! Let me at him!" I thought. "What can I do about this situation?"

I was starting to see that my mothering skills were woefully inadequate to relieve Elizabeth's suffering. I couldn't protect her from things or people like that. So I asked God to help her.

"Lord, You're here with Elizabeth all the time, especially when things like this happen. She needs You. She's weak and vulnerable. Please help her and comfort her."

During her first two days, she'd been unable to keep anything she ate or drank down. Her intense Influenza A symptoms clashed with treatment plans. I'd never seen such extreme stomach sensitivity. She had absolutely no appetite. Nevertheless, the medical staff had procedures to follow. "You have to eat!" was their mantra. Elizabeth felt increasing pressure to do what her body refused to do. A frustrating cycle of failure quickly developed. The staff was stymied.

Since the infection was in Elizabeth's lungs, I expected we'd soon hear a loose, gross-sounding, productive cough—usually a sign of healing in the lungs. This wasn't happening in her case. The problem was—there wasn't any mucus to cough up. That wasn't a good sign. Her lungs were tight. Each breath was short. Her breathing was all too quiet. Every breath was obviously painful, but each time she took a *deep* breath, it looked like she was reacting to the stab of a knife.

Matt arrived at the hospital after work the second evening. I told him about the intensifying eating dilemma. Then I left to spend time with Sarah at home. Within minutes, a food tray was delivered to Elizabeth. He decided to try spoon feeding her some red jello. He gently offered her one spoon after another with calm, encouraging words, until she'd eaten everything in the small container.

"Elizabeth ate a whole container of jello and kept it all down!" Matt exclaimed when he got home later that night.

I gasped in amazement. "That's unbelievable!"

On the third morning, her nurse made another attempt to get her medications down. They came right back up. Still meals were delivered throughout the day. Pressure to eat was applied. Elizabeth looked at me with pleading eyes that said: "I just can't do it! Help me."

By the afternoon, I pushed the medical staff to formulate a new procedure for Elizabeth—"No food." The procedure was agreed upon. A note was made in her chart. Within a couple of hours, the nursing shift changed. Another food tray was brought to her for dinner. Elizabeth ignored it.

That night, I returned to visit her after dinner. A different nurse in the night shift sensed my frustration over the food issue for Elizabeth. She joined in on the quest to find anything Elizabeth's stomach would tolerate.

"How about popsicles? Do you think she'd try them?" she asked.

Before I left for the night, I mentioned the idea to Elizabeth. She perked up a little.

"A popsicle sounds good!" she said.

That was the first thing in many days she seemed interested in eating.

The next morning, on my way into the hospital, I bought a box of popsicles. I'd felt helpless for four days, so I was excited to actually *do* something. As soon as I got to her room, I unwrapped a blue popsicle for her. I watched as she began to enjoy—really enjoy!—the first bite or two. Seeing her eat something willingly filled me with great joy.

Then I went to the nurse's desk to ask if there was a refrigerator close by where I could store the rest of the box. Two nurses heard how thrilled I was to see Elizabeth actually eating a popsicle.

"What?! Elizabeth can't have anything to eat! Her chart says, 'NO FOOD'!" said one of the nurses. The way she said it made me feel like a mother who'd just tried to poison her daughter.

I frantically ran back to Elizabeth's room. "Elizabeth, wait! You can't have that!" I said. I could see my words delivered a sad blow to her. She was so enjoying her popsicle.

"Why?" asked Elizabeth.

"A nurse said you can't have it because your chart has a "No Food" policy in it now," I said. "Oh, man, I forgot all about that. Yesterday, I pushed to make that policy so the nurses would stop trying to force solid foods on you. I'm so sorry I forgot about that."

Even though I hated seeing her so disappointed, I grabbed the popsicle from her and tossed it in the nearby sink, where it slowly melted away.

The nurse who scolded me at the desk came in right away to make sure Elizabeth wasn't still eating it.

Severe confusion and frustration screamed inside us. My brain hurt trying to make sense of everything. Seeing Elizabeth so sick was awful. The days spent in her room began to feel like mental and emotional anguish for both of us. Yet it was so much worse for her considering her unrelieved physical suffering.

The popsicle "denial" put me temporarily over the edge. My face grew hot as tears blurred my vision. I had to cry. Soon, a hospital staff person came in to calm me down. She made me feel a little better. Still, I had no idea what was going on with my daughter. Helplessness ruled the day.

I decided to call our church office to request prayer. The secretary's voice was warm and caring. I gave her a brief summary of Elizabeth's previous four days.

"Is Elizabeth improving?" she asked.

Just thinking about the answer to that question made me feel more troubled. It clarified my thoughts.

"No, she's not improving at all," I said.

It helped to share our need. I knew our church family would be praying.

Elizabeth's sister, Maggie, who was two years younger, had endured three days of college classes, work, and worrying. So had John. They got together and drove up to visit Elizabeth. Once they arrived, I gave them the gown, mask, and glove demo.

"I can't get this one finger into the glove!" said John. "Is there a bigger size?"

"I think they assume one size will fit all," I said. "They're stretchy, but maybe not stretchy enough for you. What's going on there with your finger?"

"Oh, I broke it once and it never healed right," he explained. "I'm going to need a little more time."

Maggie and I started busting up in the hall outside Elizabeth's room as we watched John. It actually helped break some of the tension I'd felt earlier. Once we made it inside her room, Elizabeth was very glad to see John and Maggie.

That evening, we had dinner reservations at a nearby Japanese restaurant to celebrate Sarah's birthday. We had a small group of family and friends planning to come. Elizabeth was the one who insisted we go to celebrate her sister's birthday when I considered postponing it. So, I went home to make some preparations.

Matt arrived as I was leaving the hospital. The doctor showed up shortly after that. He and Matt connected again.

"Her case is complex," he said. "The oral medication treatment isn't working. Her symptoms are slightly worse. I'd like to move her to the ICU for the weekend where they will keep a closer eye on her."

Matt gave his permission for the move. When he got home, he told me the doctor's update as we got ready to go out. For days, I'd hoped the doctor would give reassurance that Elizabeth would be okay, but none came.

At the restaurant that night there was a lot to watch. Unique, flavorful food was sliced, cooked, thrown, torched, and delightfully displayed before us. But I felt torn. "How was I to enjoy a party for one wonderful daughter while another precious daughter lay in a hospital bed in so much pain?" I wondered. Somehow, I was able to swallow my food, but it went down past a very heavy heart.

The servers knew we were there to celebrate Sarah's birthday, so after dinner, her waitress brought her a costume. She helped Sarah into a colorful silk Japanese kimono. When they put a black wig styled into a Japanese hairstyle on Sarah's head, she really looked authentic. Then they presented her with a special dessert singing "Happy Birthday" with loud excitement.

"She looks like an attractive Japanese young woman, don't you think?" I asked Matt. He smiled a little. When he didn't say anything, I could tell he was lost in his thoughts.

At home afterward, Sarah's friends hung out for a while. They gave her lovely gifts. Although no one said a word about it, Elizabeth's situation hung like a grey cloud over the evening. Sarah had hoped they'd stay and watch a video, but they left early. She felt dejected. Her party ended on a joyless note.

John had stayed with Elizabeth while they transferred her to the ICU. After she was settled in, they gave her pain medicine through an IV. She quickly felt much more comfortable.

The next afternoon, Matt and I had a long talk with Elizabeth's doctor in ICU. I'd been craving information for days, so I fired questions at him left and right. As bad as she felt, Elizabeth didn't seem to think her illness was too serious. She didn't appear worried. I was much more concerned. As we spoke, I must have sounded bossy to the doctor.

"This isn't *your* illness, it's Elizabeth's," he said, looking directly at me.

I suddenly felt like he was bawling me out for being a foolish, meddling mother. Stinging pain from the doctor's words and tone stabbed my heart. Tears filled my eyes once again. I tried to hide them.

In her initial isolated room, Elizabeth said she felt like no one cared about her. In her mind, they were just doing their jobs. Since her case was so complicated, she was a bother. In intensive care, we saw a dramatic increase in the level of care and attentiveness Elizabeth received. Even the atmosphere was different. The title "intensive care" perfectly described what went on there.

The medical staff had concerned, kind faces. They all knew what was going on in her case. The ICU nurses seemed to think of everything. They even cared about grooming. Once they determined it had been five days since Elizabeth had been able to wash her hair, a nurse was sensitive to that need. She washed Elizabeth's hair for her while she lay in bed. Then she let the water drain off into a huge plastic bag. We all felt thankful to have her in ICU.

During that weekend, it was encouraging to see her finally experience relief from the unrelenting pain that had been her constant companion. We couldn't help but feel relief ourselves. As we spent time with her, we loved seeing her talk and laugh more normally. We assumed Elizabeth was on the mend.

CHAPTER TWO

Something Drastic

"WOULDN'T IT BE GREAT IF Elizabeth could come home this week?" I thought during my early Monday morning drive to the hospital. As I got out of my car, I noticed the air was filled with the sweet fragrance of white roses blooming in nearby bushes. I appreciated their beauty on my way to the building. Once inside, I went to the phone in the hall outside of the ICU and called the desk to be admitted. I hoped to hear good news about her condition. She'd been in the hospital for seven days and in ICU for three.

As I walked toward Elizabeth's ICU room door, Dr. Glen Abergel came out. He was the pulmonologist on duty that week. He was of average height, early forties, with dark hair that framed his round face. I saw kindness behind his polite smile, and his eyes conveyed approachability and caring. My first impression was a good one.

After he introduced himself, his pleasant attitude shifted to a solemn one. "Elizabeth's condition started to deteriorate just before you got here," he said gravely.

"When she got up to use the bedside commode, her blood saturation level plummeted to a dangerously low level," he continued. "She's become hypoxic, which means her lungs are no longer doing their job. Medical professionals call her condition ARDS, an acronym for Acute Respiratory Distress Syndrome."

The doctor went on to explain the extreme measures they'd taken to help her. She was immediately placed on a ventilator with 100 percent oxygen support, the maximum assistance a person can tolerate.

I was stunned. "Now Elizabeth's so sick, she needs a ventilator," I thought. My mind struggled to shift gears from optimism to careful concentration as I listened to more of his negative report.

"Elizabeth's lung condition is severe," the doctor added. "We had to decrease the amount of work her body puts into the act of breathing. We also gave her medication that completely paralyzed her and put her into a drug-induced coma. Since every movement of the body uses oxygen, keeping her in a deep sleep will cut down on any unnecessary movements that would waste any of her limited oxygen supply."

Her doctor felt the paralytic medication could also provide other helpful affects. He hoped it would decrease the very high pressure in her lungs. He also thought the medication would give them better control of the ventilator.

"He can't be talking about Elizabeth!" I thought. "He's using such ominous sounding words—'deteriorate, dangerously low level, severe lung condition'. There's no encouragement in them."

My earlier hopes were crushed.

In the ICU, I suddenly found myself in a world of specialists. For starters, Dr. Abergel was a pulmonologist—a doctor who specialized in diagnosing and treating lung and respiratory tract conditions and diseases. But he was also an intensivist—a specialist in critical care.

When the doctor explained the grave trouble Elizabeth's lungs were in, he also told me how they should be functioning.

"Healthy breathing continually supplies oxygen to the blood and then to all vital organs and tissues to sustain life. The term 'blood saturation' means the amount of oxygen in the blood. A deficient amount of saturated blood could cause injury to the brain and eventually death. Healthy saturation numbers are close to 100%."

Elizabeth's numbers were nowhere near that.

Earlier that morning, my family thought Elizabeth had been improving. Maggie and Sarah had gone back to school and Matt went to work. I told the doctor I wanted to call my husband back to the hospital, so I left the ICU.

While I waited for him, I felt my own breathing quicken as fear tried to get a strong grip. During Elizabeth's first five days in the hospital, I'd already cried in front of her twice. At times, I'm quite emotional. I knew I wouldn't get through the situation if my emotions continually drained me.

Alone in the restroom, I made a downward swipe with my hand in front of a motion sensor which triggered a paper towel to release from a dispenser near the sink. This new invention distracted me briefly from the doctor's words I'd just heard. Then I suddenly felt a huge need to pray. "Oh God, please help Elizabeth. And Lord, I need you to shut off my emotions while she's here. Help me respond to this in faith."

For years prior to that day, God had been working on me to improve my reaction skills when trouble hit. I'd spent time in two extremes—either the passionate hothead or the deep, analytical thinker who dove into depression easily. As a passionate hothead, I'd let my opinions be known in a flash when problems arose. As an adult, I'd always believed it was important to say what I felt. On the other hand, when I went overboard as a deep thinker, I went into some dark, helpless places. I became paralyzed there.

The Lord had been training me to go to Him first when trouble hit. If I did, He'd help me react in faith. In 2 Corinthians 10:5 He instructs us to "take captive every thought to make it obedient to Christ." He alone knows how to draw a safe line for thoughts in my mind. The process to teach me wise restraint was still ongoing. I'd learned that He'd guide my reactions if I asked Him to.

Without God, my own ways had failed me too many times already. My words and reactions only caused damage and hurt.

"If I don't rely fully on God's wise thought control today, I know I'll be in deep trouble," I thought.

I noticed a supernatural calm began to come over me as I waited for Matt.

When Matt arrived, we met with Dr. Abergel in the waiting room. For Matt's benefit, the doctor explained Elizabeth's condition and the aggressive steps they'd taken earlier. Then he took us into ICU to show us her lung x-ray on the lighted panel. As we stared at the display, he explained that the viral infection in her lower lungs had swept into her upper lungs as well.

"Elizabeth's taken a giant turn for the worse," he said in a somber tone.

Astonished, I stood motionless. His words took my own breath away. I didn't want them to be true.

"So, if someone's lungs are full of infection, can the person breathe?" I asked. "Can this be fatal?"

"Your daughter has a fifty-fifty chance of survival," the doctor replied.

Matt let out a huge exhale as if he'd been kicked in the stomach. God kept my emotions in check, but I felt all the energy drain out of my body. Whatever Dr. Abergel said after "fifty-fifty chance" was a blur. My thinking became fixated on that phrase. I could barely pay attention to anything else.

As the doctor finished his comments, fearful thoughts stabbed each of our hearts. "I don't want to lose my daughter!" thought Matt. "She'll be robbed of her whole life."

"Elizabeth could die today," I thought, shuddering at how horrible those words sounded.

"How can we fix her?" Matt wondered.

Both of us had one common thought: "Lord, let me trade places with Elizabeth. I'd do it in a heartbeat!"

There was nothing more Dr. Abergel could tell us at that time, so he guided us back to the ICU waiting room. Our shocked bodies and minds appreciated his assistance. We sat down, continuing to grapple with Elizabeth's prognosis. I noticed my heart had begun to hurt. It felt heavy.

"What do we do now?" I asked.

"We need to call people," said Matt. "Elizabeth needs everyone's prayers."

Then we began the unpleasant task of calling family, close friends, and our church prayer chain to let them know Elizabeth's condition had become extremely critical.

While Matt was telling many people about the crisis, he had the sensation it was someone else talking on the phone, not him. "This can't be happening!" he thought. "How can I get out of this nightmare?"

The hardest call to make was to Maggie at Azusa Pacific University. When I reached her on the phone, I didn't want to scare her. God kept me calm as I spoke.

"Elizabeth's lung infection has become much worse this morning, Maggie. The doctor even said she might not make it. She has a fifty-fifty chance of survival."

Maggie gasped, but she felt confused because my words were urgent, while my voice wasn't. Once she realized my words were true, she felt overwhelmed with sorrow. Fear took hold. Hot, from-the-heart tears came so quickly, they practically jumped from her eyes. Minutes later she was in her teal-colored Jetta, unafraid to speed down the freeway to get to her sister and family that needed her.

The sixty miles separating us may as well have been a million. It was awful to be so far apart. We just wanted to hug her.

"I don't like the thought of Maggie making the Azusa to Camarillo drive while she's really upset," Matt said.

"Me either," I said. "She'll be crying and it will be hard for her to see clearly."

Yet we had no control over that, either, so we simply prayed for her safe arrival.

On the road, Maggie drove pretty much on auto pilot. Horrifying thoughts flooded her mind.

"I can't imagine Elizabeth no longer being in my life. How can I possibly take over the family role as eldest daughter and sister? If she dies, how will I live without her?"

Maggie also thought about the many things she loved about her sister. She'd always looked up to Elizabeth, admiring her excellent example of what it meant to be a good student, loving daughter, and woman of God.

She kept blinking away tears, doing her best to focus on the road.

"Will I ever get to talk to her again?" she wondered. "When I saw her two days ago, she looked much better. What happened to make her condition so critical today?"

Maggie's cell phone rang. It was John. He'd tried to call us back, but couldn't get through. She filled him in on the details from the doctor's prognosis.

"I can't believe this!" he said, shocked to hear Elizabeth had only a fifty-fifty chance. "I'm coming to the hospital, too."

Everyone we called that day was astonished to hear how quickly Elizabeth had become so ill. The news and request for serious prayer for our precious daughter spread like wildfire.

After calling Sarah at the high school, we spoke again with Dr. Abergel.

"I must say you're handling this really well," he said. "You seem quite calm."

We felt God had begun to provide His peace and strength.

"God is helping us," I said with a slight smile.

Each time we saw Dr. Abergel, he gave us more details about Elizabeth's condition. Our intensive crash course on lungs had definitely begun. We learned that healthy lungs are made up of two large, side-by-side air sacs in the chest together with the spaces which contain them. These spaces between the lung sacs and the chest walls are known as pleural cavities. Each pleural cavity is a negative pressure area which cannot contain any air.

If a lung sac develops a leak, air gets into the pleural cavity and becomes trapped. This trapped air is known as a pneumothorax. Earlier that morning before she was put on the ventilator, the tops of both of Elizabeth's lungs developed large leaks. Air became trapped in her pleural cavities. Positive pressure was then put on the lung sacs from the outside.

When a patient with lung leaks breathes in air from the ventilator, it causes additional pressure to force more air through the leak. This makes the pneumothorax grow. The integrity of the lungs becomes even more compromised. The pneumothorax eventually puts so much pressure on the lung sac, it becomes badly displaced and shrinks in size. This leads to a collapsed lung. Elizabeth's lungs had collapsed in many places. Breathing became extremely difficult.

Dr. Abergel quickly prioritized Elizabeth's multiple problems based on whether or not they were immediately life-threatening. The collapsed lungs became the first priority. They had to be re-inflated. He called on a thoracic surgeon from Camarillo's parent hospital, St. John's Regional Medical Center in Oxnard, to insert two large chest tubes into her pleural cavities. He put one under each arm in the upper rib cage to relieve the pressure. These tubes began to drain excess air from the pleural cavities.

They also allowed the lungs to re-inflate and prevented further air from accumulating.

"The procedure went well, said Dr. Abergel. "Every procedure attempted at this point has to. With so many things seriously wrong with her lungs, there's no room for error."

Elizabeth began receiving intensive care from highly trained and skilled infectious disease doctors, nurses, and respiratory therapists.

The infectious disease doctor passionately began the search for the exact virus causing Elizabeth's infection. Her blood was tested for anything suspected as a source including Legionnaires' disease, tuberculosis, SARS, and Valley Fever. All her test results came back negative. The doctors remained stumped. Since they hadn't pinpointed a definite illness, Elizabeth remained potentially contagious. We were still required to wear the isolation garb when we were in her room.

Then the infectious disease doctor suggested an open-lung biopsy to help discover the facts. The procedure required surgery to obtain a lung tissue sample that would later be examined under a microscope for cancer, infection, or lung disease. If they knew what virus they faced, it would make it much easier to treat.

"Elizabeth wouldn't survive the procedure, so it's not an option," Dr. Abergel responded.

When I heard the doctor attach the possibility of death to my daughter's name, it seemed unbelievable to me. The words were chilling. It stirred the parental pain swirling around in my heart.

"This is so serious! This is so sad. What's going to happen to my Elizabeth?" I wondered.

Throughout my Christian life, I'd wondered how people got through a terrifying period of crisis with their faith intact. I'd heard stories about others who walked in faith when their worst nightmare happened or when the bottom dropped out of their lives.

"How can they feel secure when everything that made up life as they knew it disappeared?" I asked myself.

I knew I wanted to be a believer with that kind of faith.

"But, how did they do it?" I wondered.

As we began our journey through Elizabeth's health crisis, the Lord started to show us how.

Some out-of-town relatives wanted to come to the hospital, but we weren't sure what the day would hold. We felt we needed to stay available to Elizabeth and the doctor. We didn't want to feel responsible for a large group of people. So we encouraged everyone to pray for now and wait until later to come. The truth was, we didn't know how much we needed God's people—fellow believers in Christ—but God knew. As soon as friends in town found out about Elizabeth, they began coming to the ICU waiting room to stand by us. God prompted His people to show His love and care and they sprang into action.

For example, Tami. When she heard Elizabeth had become so sick, God stirred her deeply and vigorously. She made a beeline for me.

When Tami walked in, she seemed intently focused as God's delivery agent. She handed me a pretty bag which held a gift and a note. She immediately encouraged me to see what was in the bag. I took a beautiful Russian mohair shawl and the note out of the bag. Tami lovingly helped drape the shawl over my shoulders. The soft, lightweight shawl and the accompanying note reminded me of the soft and gentle touch of the Master's hand on my life that day.

Tami included applicable Bible verses in her note. She knew I needed to hear the Lord's voice that day. I needed to look at things from His perspective.

"There's no doubt the Lord has everything under control," Tami said confidently. "He has purposes for this situation. What's happening with Elizabeth is no random mistake that God knows nothing about."

I thanked Tami for her gift as tears welled up in my eyes. The Lord sent this dear woman, the shawl, and His own encouraging words to strengthen and comfort my heart.

I'd always liked Tami. We'd met around ten years earlier in a small town about a half hour from Camarillo. We both had three young daughters of similar ages. From time to time, they were involved in the same activities, which gave us opportunities to talk. Somehow, the Lord always became the main topic of conversation. Her passion for the Lord, His Word, His will and His ways made a deep impression on me every time.

Over the years, both of our families moved to Camarillo. Recently, our paths hadn't crossed very often. So, Matt and I wondered how she'd found out about Elizabeth's condition. We discovered the communication link that ultimately reached her had started with my brother-in-law. He told his brother, who told his wife, who called Tami. In no time, the information passed between three separate cities in Southern California. News about Elizabeth's condition continued to spread rapidly, anywhere someone knew her or our family.

Later, as I glanced at the verses I'd been given, one scripture stood out and offered an immediate explanation for our situation.

> "Consider it pure joy, my brothers, whenever you face trials of many kinds, because you know that the testing of your faith develops perseverance. Perseverance must finish its work so that you may be mature and complete, not lacking anything" (James 1:2–4).

I kept reading the verses Tami brought me. Another portion of scripture particularly grabbed my heart.

> "My grace is sufficient for you, for my power is made perfect in weakness. Therefore I will boast all the more gladly about my weaknesses, so that Christ's power may rest on me. That is why, for Christ's sake, I delight in weaknesses, in insults, in hardships, in persecutions, in difficulties. For when I am weak, then I am strong" (2 Corinthians 12:9–10).

He promised He would give us His powerful strength to face whatever was ahead. I thought for a while about that.

"Lord, I need your power in me now more than ever," I prayed. "May your very power rest on me."

I suddenly realized the developments of the morning put Matt and I on the same page spiritually for the first time. Each of us was a hurting parent who desperately wanted God to save their daughter. We were utterly dependent on Him.

Still, we were unaccustomed to sharing God's personal work in our lives together. Generally, Matt was not a very talkative, expressive man. He'd usually kept his deeper emotions in check. At times, he was withdrawn. Sometimes during the months of spring, our individual schedules were so full that we neglected each other. We'd been in "neglect mode" for a few weeks before Elizabeth became sick.

However, we'd been married close to twenty-five years and we could read each other pretty well. With so much on our minds that morning, we found words between us weren't always necessary. We could tell by looking at each other that we felt the same way. One time, we slowed down enough to notice each other and Matt took my hand briefly. Just being close had a somewhat calming effect as we faced the uncertain hours ahead.

"I'm glad I'm not alone in this," I said.

"Me too," Matt said.

Matt and I discovered a little prayer chapel near the ICU entrance. When we went inside, we noticed the lights were dim and it was quiet there. There were small pews to sit on. Near the front of the room, a large opened Bible rested on a small podium. I picked up a book that was sitting in a rack on the wall. I looked inside it and read a few prayer requests people had written.

The room itself seemed to whisper: "Come, lay your burden down."

We thought we'd be able to talk privately there with Maggie and Sarah when they arrived.

They arrived mid-afternoon at the same time. As soon as we saw them, Matt and I each hugged a daughter and held on tight while tears fell.

"I don't want Elizabeth to die!" cried Sarah.

"How can this be happening?" asked Maggie.

Matt guided our family into the prayer chapel. It felt good to be together. We told our daughters all we knew at that time. Then we unloaded our burden for Elizabeth together.

"Oh Lord, please heal Elizabeth's lungs."

"Please help her now."

"We ask you to guide her doctor. Give him your wisdom."

"Lord, we don't want Elizabeth to die. We love her so much. Please heal her body."

As a family team, we united to face the crisis together. We hugged each other again as more tears fell.

Then, Matt took them into Elizabeth's room one by one. When they first saw their sister, they just stared at her. It was hard for them to see her so sick. A nurse told them to talk to Elizabeth because, even though she was in a deep sleep, she could hear their voices and sense they were near.

Maggie took her words to heart.

"Hi, Elizabeth! It's Maggie. I'm sorry you're so sick. I really love you. We're all praying for you. Be strong," she said.

Sarah followed the nurse's recommendation, too.

"Hi, Elizabeth!" It's Sarah. I'm here. I love you. I hope you get well soon."

Meanwhile, a waiting room corner began to fill with Elizabeth's classmates and local friends who cared deeply about her. John and his mom were among them.

Nothing would keep my sister, Jeri, away from the hospital that day. The minute she heard Elizabeth's condition had become so critical, she explained it to her employer.

"I'm outta here!" she said.

We weren't sure she needed to come, but she had no doubt. She battled Orange County afternoon freeway traffic, which made the usually two-hour drive much longer.

Jeri, a strong, faithful woman, has courageously suffered loss many times in her own life, which has made her a compassionate and tender soul. She can sense when someone's hurting or in a crisis. She'll come alongside, gently place her strong hand on them, and pray.

When she arrived in the crowded waiting room, her face said it all—"This must be awful. I'm here for you." In our time of trouble, she listened and stayed nearby. She seemed to know what to say and what not to say—toughness and gentleness combined. She'd raised two football players, which probably helped her become both a sweet and tough "cookie." Her supportive presence with us spoke volumes. I felt stronger with her there. I knew her prayers for Elizabeth were unceasing.

Church friends, Tim and Laurie, had also arrived, offering their comfort and support. Tim was an elder at our church. He was also a medical doctor. Toward late afternoon, I had a request for him. I looked for a moment to talk with him alone.

"Can you arrange to have the elders come tonight to lay hands on Elizabeth, anoint her with oil, and pray for God to heal her, if we feel she needs it?" I asked.

"I'd be happy to," Tim answered.

CHAPTER THREE

God's Place of Refuge

MANY HAD GATHERED WITH US in the waiting room from both near and far. We hadn't had an update from the doctor for hours. As one, we felt the heavy weight of Elizabeth's unfavorable odds.

Then the Holy Spirit prompted us to obey Hebrews 4:16:

> "Let us then approach the throne of grace with confidence, so that we may receive mercy and find grace to help us in our time of need."

With our collective humanness screaming internally, "I'm so afraid," I suggested we pray. Together as believers we entered God's presence on Elizabeth's behalf. Age and church affiliation were of no importance. Anyone who wanted to could pray, and in the pauses between prayers, individuals read scriptures God brought to mind. In no time, the Lord began to speak faith and hope into our hearts.

After a while, Matt read a verse, Isaiah 49:15–16:

> "Can a mother forget the baby at her breast and have no compassion on the…"

He choked up, unable to go on. After a slight pause, he continued as his voice quivered,

> "...no compassion on the child she has borne? Though she may forget, I will not forget you! See, I have engraved you on the palms of my hands; your walls are ever before me."

I was surprised, but impressed to see him participate. He hadn't jumped in like that too often before.

Our daughters had never seen their father cry. His new vulnerability scared Maggie.

"Dad has always seemed so strong, but right now, he knows there's nothing he can do to fix this," thought Maggie. "He doesn't know what will happen. If Dad looks upset, this is a big deal!"

As Maggie and Sarah both heard how intensely he petitioned God for Elizabeth, they began to cry, too. They'd also never seen him so focused on prayer and so comfortable praying in public.

After a few more prayers, someone boldly read a verse:

> "You will keep in perfect peace him whose mind is steadfast, because he trusts in you" (Isaiah 26:3).

The Lord inspired the reading of many magnificent verses. In those blessed moments, as we shared together, the Holy Spirit within us began to gently whisper with a powerful grace greater than our fear.

Calm down. I'm with you. Receive My peace.

Other believers who'd arrived in the waiting room after we'd started, joined in and prayed, too. The unity within the Body of Christ drew them right in. By His Spirit we sensed His presence among us. He'd transformed a waiting room into a prayer chapel. That precious, powerful time lasted quite a while.

God had a multifaceted answer to my earlier question—"How do believers get through a terrifying crisis with their faith intact?" In addition to receiving the love and support of the Body of Christ, He began to reveal another aspect—His place of refuge. He wanted us to come and stay there.

He'd just prompted us to pray fervently—one of the amazing activities that transports us by faith into His presence—our place of refuge. Scripture tells us we may receive what we need during a crisis from a person, God Himself.

> "God is our refuge and strength, an ever-present help in trouble" (Psalm 46:1).

Many Psalms and other scriptures use descriptive phrases for God's amazing place of refuge such as: "under His wings", "in the cleft of the rock", "my hiding place", "in the shadow of the Almighty", "a shelter in the storm", and "a path through many waters."

In God's presence, His people find stability, tranquility, and His many gracious benefits. God's place of refuge is so lovely! In it, as sheep, we can lie down in green pastures and be led by quiet waters. As His children, He carries us and holds us by His right hand. He makes our heavy burdens light and enables us by faith to soar on wings like eagles. He prevents us from falling and He has promised never to desert or forsake us. And lastly, He is committed to ministering to each of us individually, satisfying our needs.

The Lord is confident in the refuge He provides. He says,

> "Taste and see that the Lord is good; blessed is the man who takes refuge in Him" (Psalm 34:8).

As we prayed, the Spirit within the Body of Christ also naturally guided us into another amazing activity God used to keep us going to Him for refuge—reading and meditating on His Word. I'd begun noticing God's place of refuge possesses an unusual quietness amidst chaos. He wanted us to listen carefully to Him. That day He impressed His words on me more deeply than I'd ever experienced before.

We realized God was reiterating what we'd been learning for many years in church about His Word—that it is incredibly powerful and authoritative. He sends it into our hearts to make things different. Psalm 19:7–8 describes some of the active agents in God's Word this way:

> "The law of the Lord is perfect, reviving the soul. The statutes of the Lord are trustworthy, making wise the

simple. The precepts of the Lord are right, giving joy to
the heart. The commands of the Lord are radiant, giving
light to the eyes."

His Spirit was prompting our spirits to learn His ways through His Word. We were just starting to see that the Lord actually teaches some of His most profound faith lessons in the quiet refuge He provides during times of crisis.

I had so much on my mind, yet the Lord continued to clearly communicate what He knew I needed to hear. It was unbelievable! At that time, He reminded me of a quote from C.H. Spurgeon that stood out to me from my college years. It was spoken over a century ago on Jan. 7, 1855, when Spurgeon was only twenty years old. Recommending the consolatory aspects of meditating on God, he said:

> "Oh, there is, in contemplating Christ, a balm for every wound; in musing on the Father, there is a quietus for every grief; and in the influence of the Holy Ghost, there is a balsam for every sore. Would you lose your sorrow? Would you drown your cares? Then go, plunge yourself in the Godhead's deepest sea; be lost in His immensity; and you shall come forth as from a couch of rest, refreshed and invigorated. I know nothing which can so comfort the soul; so calm the swelling billows of sorrow and grief; so speak peace to the winds of trial, as a devout musing upon the subject of the Godhead."[3]

God's Word presented us with perfect truths to contemplate.

So much happens when we open a Bible and unhurriedly think on truth. When we do, truth connects with the Holy Spirit indwelling us. The Spirit longs to see obedience to truth in believers, so He gives us godly desires, abilities, and motivation in that direction. With each truth we

---

3   J.I. Packer, <u>Knowing God</u> © 1973 by InterVarsity Press: Downers Grove, Illinois #14—In the English language only for distribution in the USA and Philippines only. Reproduced by permission of Hodder and Stoughton Limited, London. Territories granted: World excluding the USA and dependencies, and the Philippine Republic.

embraced, He touched and changed our hearts and minds. He exchanged our thoughts for His thoughts. We began to react in God's ways.

―――

Since God's supply of help for us was so abundant, I began to wonder—"How do unbelievers get through a terrifying crisis like ours by themselves?"

Perhaps this is where you find yourself. Maybe you're also going through a crisis right now, or you've been through crises in the past. You realize you don't personally know this amazingly helpful God, but you want to know Him.

For this to happen, you must understand two basic facts. First, God is holy—completely pure, loving, and worthy of worship. He created every person to reflect His beauty and live His way. But the second basic fact—man is sinful—makes this impossible without a willing acceptance of His help. You may believe the notion that only the worst people sin. But every person is born into sin. In fact, it's our nature. It's a deceiving, despicable trap and it's the worst trouble people face.

In the Bible, God tells us that on their own, there isn't any righteous person who does good and seeks Him, not even one. Many in our society aren't too familiar with the word sin. But God's perspective on it is clear. Here's one list of specific sins, among many, in the Bible to help us know what it is.

> "People will be lovers of themselves, lovers of money, boastful, proud, abusive, disobedient to their parents, ungrateful, unholy, without love, unforgiving, slanderous, without self-control, brutal, not lovers of the good, treacherous, rash, conceited, lovers of pleasure rather than lovers of God—having a form of godliness but denying its power" (2 Timothy 3:2–5a).

Our sin indeed separates us from a holy God who deeply desires to share a loving relationship with us. He determined that a sinless, pure sacrifice be made to pay the penalty for sin. We can't pay the penalty for our own sin—only Jesus could. He alone is able to forgive our sin and bring us to God.

In His great love, God provides everything we need to rescue us from our trouble. Jesus Christ, God's sinless Son, came and died on the cross for our sin, was buried, and raised to life on the third day.

Placing our faith in Jesus also gives us eternal life. Our relationship with God begins there. It's all a lavish gift from God.

God is reaching out to you today. He invites you to believe what He's done for you, to receive Him, and commit your life to Him.

In the Bible God tells us the next step to take.

> "That if you confess with your mouth, 'Jesus is Lord,' and believe in your heart that God raised Him from the dead, you will be saved. For it is with your heart that you believe and are justified, and it is with your mouth that you confess and are saved" (Romans 10:9–10).

It's actually quite simple. If you are ready to trust Jesus right now, you can talk to God and pray something like this:

"God, up until now, I've lived my life without You. I have sinned against You. I have many troubles in my life, but I never understood sin was my biggest trouble. I need You. I don't want to handle things on my own anymore.

"Jesus, please forgive me. I believe you died on the cross to pay for my sins. I believe you rose from the dead. Thank you for loving me. I give my life to You. Please teach me how to live in Your good ways and to experience Your help all the rest of my life."

Our God had been working powerfully in our hearts, revealing one phase of His help after another. However, by late afternoon, the sense of danger surrounding Elizabeth's situation began grabbing at us forcefully again. Remaining in God's place of refuge was harder than it sounded. Temptation to leave came often. I felt I was in a tug-of-war. When I drew near to God, I felt peace and safety. If I gave in to fear even briefly, I opened the floodgate of more fearful thoughts which could multiply rapidly.

When the next wave of fear washed over me, my Ever-Present Help saw my weakness. He drew near to provide more of what He alone could supply. Each time my need increased, His supply increased as well.

That day I actually felt like a one-year-old child who'd fallen and received an ugly gash in her forehead. The wound was bleeding excessively and I was crying wildly. My dad picked me up in his arms immediately. My mom brought some gauze bandages to try to slow the bleeding and cover the gash as they rushed me to the doctor's office. They were sure I'd need stitches so I would heal properly.

My dad knew the shot to numb the injured area would hurt me. He also knew just the sight of a needle coming at me would terrify me. Until he had to put me down, he held me more tightly than ever before.

When he had to lay me down on a table so the doctor could work, he got his face as close to mine as he could. He kept my attention on him and his voice. His calm, loving voice constantly whispered tender words of reassurance. He stayed close so I couldn't see everything that was happening to me.

After a little while, the doctor asked my dad to move out of the way so he could put in the stitches. My dad found another position. He went behind my head and placed His strong arms on top of my shoulders. He was prepared to hold me still in case I tried to squirm away from the doctor. He continued to speak loving, encouraging words near my face all through the ordeal. He gave all he had to get me through the worst of it.

Our God is the same way—He loves us enough to get right in our faces when we need Him most, if we let Him.

His words of assurance to my heart that afternoon did not come audibly, but directly, concisely, and with authority. They spoke of additional help He was sending.

Diane, on your own, you have no strength to face what's ahead, so I'll give you Mine.

He performed a "spiritual exchange" in me. He substituted my complete fear, anxiety, and weakness for His faith, hope, and courage. Up until that time, I'd never felt so strong in Him. My inadequacy drained out and His adequacy flooded in to replace it. I didn't even feel like myself. I sensed His power in me and He assured me it would be fully adequate for whatever I'd face.

I wasn't the only one to feel that way—God had begun to make my whole family unusually strong in Him. We'd never been more beautiful. God's strength enabled us to exhibit His beautiful traits, not our own. I marveled at that kind of strength, the kind which makes no sense as the world sees it.

As I considered the strength of God, He whispered a scripture passage to my heart again that I'd read earlier in Tami's note:

"My grace is sufficient for you, for my power is made perfect in weakness. Therefore I will boast all the more gladly about my weaknesses, so that Christ's power may rest on me. That is why, for Christ's sake, I delight in weaknesses, in insults, in hardships, in persecutions, in difficulties. For when I am weak, then I am strong" (2 Corinthians 12:9–10).

I realized God had just infused Christ's power into me.

We didn't know that while Elizabeth was fighting for her life, three other people were doing the same in ICU beds nearby. As we waited through many long hours in the waiting room, we began to learn how the ICU system works. We started to become familiar with hospital terminology. Matt and I panicked when we heard "Code Blue—ICU Number 157" over the hospital's loud speaker. We knew what "code blue" meant from television shows—a patient requires immediate resuscitation—but we didn't know Elizabeth's room number. We looked at each other.

"Is 157 Elizabeth's room number?" Matt asked in alarm.

"I don't remember even seeing a number on her door," I said. "I have no idea!"

The hospital chaplain happened to be nearby. He seemed to sense our anxiety because he ran over to us.

"Number 157 isn't Elizabeth's room number," he said.

We were relieved!

A little later, the chaplain came back to us.

"I was just in ICU. I overheard the medical staff say Elizabeth's procedure had gone well," he said. "Elizabeth is much better."

We felt overjoyed.

"But, why is the chaplain giving us a medical report?" I wondered. "Why aren't we hearing this from her doctor?"

At that point, Tim and Laurie looked around at all the college students and friends who'd assembled. They picked up on the much lighter mood after the chaplain's report and left to order pizza. Before they returned, however, we saw the doctor again. We told him what the chaplain had said.

"No, I'm sorry," he said, shaking his head. "Elizabeth is still gravely ill."

By then, McGovern supporters dominated the waiting room. I got their attention and relayed the doctor's report. So we began another prayer and scripture reading session. When Tim and Laurie came back with pizza, they could tell the atmosphere of the room had resumed the serious, burdened mood we'd shared earlier. Tim quietly put the pizza down on the table while we prayed, and slipped out to contact the elders. He felt sure it was time for them to come anoint Elizabeth and pray for her.

To prepare the way for the elders to pray, I asked the nurse if we could have a large group of 12 or so in Elizabeth's room all at once. The infectious disease doctor standing nearby overheard my question.

"We'll help make it work," she said.

Shortly before seven o'clock, elders from our church began to gather in the hall outside the waiting room. A nurse wheeled the cabinet containing disposable gowns, masks, and gloves into the hall. Matt stood in front of the men and demonstrated how to suit up.

John had brought some anointing oil with myrrh with him. He wanted to anoint Elizabeth, too, so he got ready to go in with the elders. A few moments later, all the men were lined up near the ICU entrance, ready to go.

Jeri felt comforted when these godly men in their yellow gowns quietly filed into ICU.

"It feels like Jesus has just entered the building, and He's going to take care of Elizabeth," she whispered as she leaned toward Maggie and Sarah.

The group pretty much filled what little space remained in Elizabeth's crowded room, which contained many vital pieces of equipment. One monitor tracked her blood saturation level and heart rate. A cuff on her arm routinely checked her blood pressure. A steel IV stand near her bed held bags of liquid connected to the IV line, which delivered necessary fluids and medication to Elizabeth's system. We saw the ventilator tube going down her throat and heard its steady, mechanical inhales and exhales. It was also monitoring the respiratory rates and pressures in her lungs.

She remained asleep. The light over her bed softly illuminated her face and revealed the truth: We were about to pray for a very sick person. As I stood near my daughter, I felt weak and helpless, aware I could do nothing in my own strength to help her. Her illness seemed monstrous.

"If God doesn't help her, she won't make it," I thought.

The pastor stood opposite Matt and me, near Elizabeth's head. Just before the elders began to pray, he dabbed oil from a small jar on his finger, reached up, and put it on her forehead. John stood next to the pastor. He took a small portion of oil from his little bottle, stepped up, and anointed Elizabeth as well. Then the men began to pray—prayer after faithful prayer lifted to the throne of grace. I knew there was nothing greater we could do. Righteous men united in prayer is scriptural and beautiful. God calls their prayers powerful and effective.

After they finished praying, they each put their isolation garb in the "discard" container in Elizabeth's room on the way out. Then they quietly left ICU and joined the crowd in the waiting room, which now spilled into the hall.

Just after Matt and I left Elizabeth's room, a nurse stopped us and asked us if we wanted to hear something exciting.

"Sure!" we both said.

"While the men prayed for Elizabeth, we saw her blood saturation level go up to 93! It hasn't done that all day!" she said. "The acceptable level in her case is 80—she's been in the 80's throughout the day. All of us at the nurses' station were so excited to see the numbers change on the monitor!"

When we left the ICU, we discovered a group of her friends was preparing to go in to pray. Some of these young people had fond memories of Elizabeth loving poor people during mission trips to Mexico, sensing God's sovereign plan in a Bible study on the book of Revelation, and faithfully praying for them as they relied on the Lord to survive the pressures of high school. Her newer friends shared the joys of the Biola community with her. All of these friends easily saw who Elizabeth was in

Christ. They each knew her as a person who was willing to let her God use her life any way He wanted to—no matter what.

As they prepared for their visit, the Holy Spirit whispered to me.

There's a worship band among this group. Ask their leader to start the group singing after they pray.

"What? You want us to sing in Elizabeth's room now, Lord?" I asked.

That's exactly what I want, God responded.

"Lord, I don't know if we can. How do we sing at a time like this?" I asked.

I had to think for a moment. While I considered the idea, the face of a mature believer popped into my head. I remembered the time she told me that when it's dark and bad, that's the best time to praise God! She believed it didn't matter if praising God seemed radical or ridiculous.

Step out in faith. I'll enable you. Start with "Blessed Be The Name of the Lord".

"Oh, that's a good one, Lord!" I told Him, warming a little to His suggestion.

I loved that song the first time I heard it. I'd sung it with gusto many times before Elizabeth got sick. The words in the song talk about God's name being blessed in "the land that is plentiful" where "streams of abundance flow," as well as times "in the desert place" and "on the road marked with suffering."[4]

"But Lord, singing when someone may die?" I asked.

I needed to ask myself a couple of questions.

"Did you really mean what you sang before or were you just mouthing words? Is your faith and love for God deep enough to actually sing and bless Him at this time?"

The more I thought about it, the stronger the desire to sing became. God made it seem like the right thing to do.

Before the new group entered the ICU, I asked the worship leader to lead the group in praise songs after we prayed. He agreed to do so.

Once again, beautiful, faithful prayers filled Elizabeth's room.

---

4   "Blessed Be Your Name", words and music by Matt and Beth Redman, © 2002. Thankyou Music(PRS) (adm. worldwide at EMICMGPublishing.com excluding Europe which is adm. By Kingswaysongs). All rights reserved. Used by permission.

"Dear Father, we ask you to touch Elizabeth with your healing power."

"Lord Jesus, we pray You'll heal her sick lungs."

"Please bring Elizabeth back to us."

"Lord, please give her body Your strength to recover."

"Thank you for holding Elizabeth in Your hands."

Later, as we sang together, the Lord worked to shift our focus from Elizabeth's gigantic need onto Himself.

I'm the only One who can meet her need, He whispered to me between songs. *Keep your eyes on Me.*

While we sang, I sensed a strange, wonderful unity with Elizabeth. Even though she was asleep, I believed she heard us and worshipped God with us in spirit.

When we returned to the waiting room, it was still packed with people. Even more friends had come. One new friend was among them. I loved her faith and her tender yet bold love for the Lord. I'd felt drawn to her spirit from our first meeting. I'd heard her own daughter died suddenly two years earlier. I selfishly hoped the Lord hadn't drawn me to her because He knew I'd share the same experience.

She didn't say much; she didn't need to. When I'd first heard the words "fifty-fifty chance" hours ago, my body had tensed up. I wasn't aware of it, but my friend had a clue. She silently moved behind me and began to rub my tired shoulders. Then with a look of deep compassion, she handed me a verse to read that God had already brought to my mind twice throughout the day. I guess He really wanted me to get this message:

"My grace [My favor and loving-kindness and mercy] is enough for you [**sufficient against any danger and enables you to bear the trouble manfully**]; for My strength and power are made perfect [*fulfilled and completed*] and show themselves most effective in [*your*] weakness. Therefore, I will all the more gladly glory in my weaknesses and infirmities, that the strength and power of Christ [the Messiah] may rest [*yes, may pitch a tent over and dwell*] upon me!" (2 Corinthians 12:9, (Amplified Bible, emphasis mine).

The Lord had stirred the hearts of so many people into beautiful acts of love and support throughout that day. They each felt like ministering angels. After a while, these people began to say their "goodnights" and pledge more offers to help.

Eventually, the huge group shrank down to our immediate family and John. Matt and I wanted to stay with Elizabeth.

"Why don't you guys go home and get some sleep?" I asked Maggie, Sarah, and John. "We're going to stay in Elizabeth's room tonight," I said.

It didn't take much to convince them.

A special story ran through John's mind on the way to our house. When they got home, Sarah went straight to her room to get ready for bed. Maggie got busy on the computer.

Before he found a place to sleep, John had a question for Maggie and Sarah. "Do you want to hear a bedtime story?" he asked.

"Okay!" said Sarah.

"Let's hear it, John," said Maggie, looking away from the computer for a second.

Since both Maggie and Sarah could multi-task, they each continued doing what they were doing before. John laid down on the floor where they'd hear him well. He began telling a story about a married woman who'd just become pregnant.

"She was way past the typical age to have a baby when her doctor told her she was pregnant. It wasn't long before she became very sick and weak. Her symptoms were well beyond the normal discomforts of early pregnancy. Because of her age and increasingly poor health, her pregnancy was considered high-risk.

"The number of doctors and women embracing abortion in those days was increasing wildly. Since she was having so much difficulty, her doctors and just about everyone else actually recommended she have an abortion.

"But abortion was not easy for her to consider. She believed every baby was a gift from God. She'd begun loving the baby growing inside her when she first heard she was pregnant. At that time, the Lord drew her to Psalm 139 to give her direction and comfort. Every night she'd read it, both silently for her sake and aloud for her baby to hear. It filled her mind with thoughts of God's hands personally creating, knitting, and weaving a new human being inside her. Every day she read the passage, she'd decide not to terminate the pregnancy THAT day. She told herself she'd wait until the next day to make her final decision about abortion.

"The Psalm literally pulled her from one day to the next. As she continued to read and ponder those verses, the window she had for an abortion closed. God's words in her heart helped her resist her doctor's persistent recommendation. She was determined to persevere through the pregnancy and do all she could to protect her baby. Earlier, she'd been warned that her overall health could decline as a result of the pregnancy. But she'd come to know she could never agree to cause her baby any harm no matter how high the risk or how many physical consequences she'd encounter.

"Other physical difficulties developed in her fifth month of pregnancy requiring major abdominal surgery. God carried her safely through that surgery. Then she endured more months of poor health and weakness. After nine months and a safe labor and delivery, a healthy baby boy was born.

"Afterwards, in the delivery room, the nurse brought in the umbilical cord on a stainless steel tray. She went on at great length about the huge knot in the cord. It probably happened when the baby was small and he had freedom to move and loop a knot like that. The nurse insisted the woman was very lucky to have a live baby. She learned that if the knot had tightened during the pregnancy or delivery, it could have taken the baby's life. But God kept the knot loose. He protected both her and her baby all those months."

When the story ended, John asked, "Who do you think the baby was?"

"I have no idea," said Sarah.

"John, the baby was probably you," said Maggie.

"Yup," John said, "it was!"

John picked the perfect time to share his beautiful story of how God protected his own life. It helped calm my tired, worried daughters. When the three of them were finally settled in for the night in separate rooms and the house grew quiet, the girls took turns lovingly calling out: "Good night, John" before they closed their eyes. They both felt safe with him there that night.

CHAPTER FOUR

God At Work

BACK AT THE HOSPITAL, I still felt a little nervous to be near Elizabeth in such a critical state, but I knew I had no choice. "Because I love her, I must be with her just the way she is," I thought.

While Matt and I suited up, her nurse gave us various instructions.

"Remain quiet—no talking allowed. Don't do anything to disturb her. It's unwise to stare at her monitor numbers—it can make you crazy," she warned.

The "things we *could* do" list had only one item on it: We were allowed to hold her hands. So when we entered her room, we went to opposite sides of her bed. We each gently picked up a very warm, feverish hand. Because we vowed to remain silent and we wore the masks, we could only communicate with our eyes, a point with a finger, or by a head-jerk toward something we wanted the other to notice.

The ventilator had helped save Elizabeth's life that day. But two dangerous extremes surrounded her even while on the ventilator. The first extreme occurs when a patient receives 100 percent pure oxygen longer than the acceptable, limited time period—24 hours. After that, it becomes toxic in a human body. If the patient receives it after the 24-hour deadline, oxygen poisoning, permanent scarring, and limited future lung capacity would result. The second extreme could occur if a patient continually fails to get enough oxygen. The result is a high risk of heart attack and stroke.

The doctor told us the goal for the next two days or so.

"Elizabeth's lungs must improve and begin to saturate her blood on her own. Only then can we lower the ventilator oxygen support to 50 percent where these dangers become minimal."

If Elizabeth was awake, she'd be shocked over the abundance of help she was receiving. She'd rarely been in the position of needing a lot of help. She was always willing to give help to others.

Even as a young child, she was often on the lookout for ways she could help me. When Elizabeth was two years old and I was eight months pregnant with Maggie, I was getting dressed for church. When I dressed up, I wore flat-heeled shoes. Each shoe had a little decorative tassel on the top of it. Elizabeth had heard me complain before if a tassel got stuck inside my shoe instead of lying outside on top of it. She knew it bugged me a lot. So when I'd get dressed and put my shoes on, Elizabeth began posting herself at my feet checking on my shoe tassels. As I slipped each foot into a shoe, she would carefully pull the tassel on the outside and hold it in the proper place for me. The dreaded tassel problem was avoided.

Elizabeth's helpful heart grew through childhood. I remembered another shoe story her Grandma Mac had told us. Elizabeth was 7 or 8 years old. The story began with a walk on a gravel path along a dry river bank near our home after a Thanksgiving dinner. Elizabeth walked next to her grandma. Not long after we started our walk, a small gravel piece got into Grandma Mac's shoe. It quickly began to bother her. She knew she had to get it out right away.

Out in the open, Grandma Mac couldn't find anything to lean against while she stood on one leg to clear the gravel out. She noticed Elizabeth nearby, so she asked her if she could lean on her shoulder for a few minutes. Elizabeth eagerly offered her assistance. Her grandma got the gravel out. Soon she was good to go again. She thanked Elizabeth for her help.

After we returned home, Elizabeth told her, "Grandma, you can lean on my shoulders any time you need to."

Her grandma loved that! As a child, Elizabeth showed the deep love toward her family she still showed as a young woman. The story remains a grandmother's fond memory.

My mind snapped back to the present where it was all too clear that our precious daughter needed all the help she could get.

Earlier, we'd rejoiced at the news that Elizabeth's saturation level had gone up during the elders' prayer time over her bed. But it had gone back below 90 a while after they left her room. As Matt and I began our nighttime vigil with Elizabeth, her saturation numbers were a low 87/88, even on 100 percent oxygen support.

We began praying silently at Elizabeth's bedside. Between prayers, I had plenty of time to think.

"It's so important for Elizabeth to get off the 100 percent oxygen support within 24 hours or so," I thought. "And over 12 of the 24 hours have already passed with no lasting improvement. It seems impossible for her to make progress, but if the number went up when the elders were praying, maybe…"

Just then the Holy Spirit whispered: *Pray for her saturation number to increase.*

I thought about God's prayer request and decided to obey Him.

"Dear God, please enable Elizabeth's lungs to function well. I pray you'll move her saturation number up to an 89." I started to watch the monitor, unafraid to risk the craziness-danger the nurse mentioned earlier. Nothing happened right away.

I continued to ask God for the number to increase. "Help her move to 89. Please make her lungs stronger." I quietly prayed and prayed.

Soon, I saw an 89, then an 88, an 89, 88, 87, 88. Then it moved back to 89 and stayed there! I saw progress! I felt so excited! I joyfully thanked God for His answer to my prayers.

Then the Holy Spirit prompted me again. *Now pray for a 90.*

"That sounds like a huge jump for Elizabeth!" I thought. Even so, I began to pray again.

"Lord, please strengthen her lungs so she can saturate well at 90. Please move her number to a 90. You have the power to do what Elizabeth's body can't do on its own." After a while, I checked the monitor. The Lord did it! It was at 90! I stared at the monitor in amazement and the number fluctuated the way it had before: 90, 89, 90, 88, 90, 89. Then it moved back to 90 and remained there.

Matt saw it too. That's when our eyes really began to communicate. We were both wide-eyed with delight.

I felt a little like Abraham when he prayed to God about His plans to destroy Sodom and Gomorrah. Abraham asked if God would still destroy the wicked cities if there were 50 righteous people in them. When God said no, Abraham lowered the number and asked God if He would destroy the cities if there were 45 righteous people in them. At each no, Abraham continued to test the depth of God's mercy (within His justice) all the way down to, "What if only ten can be found there?"

Now, like Abraham, I continued to ask God for a gracious, favorable number progression. "Ninety-one, Lord—please strengthen Elizabeth's lungs to breathe and saturate well at ninety-one." Again, nothing happened immediately. But I persevered with my prayers, and some time later a 91 appeared on the monitor.

Matt had smiling eyes, and I'm sure I did too, as we continued to watch and pray.

Next, I felt bold enough to ask for a 92. It seemed like such a high number, but I asked anyway. Pretty soon the 91 changed to a 92! Tears flooded my eyes. I couldn't believe that 92! I was thrilled! The number 92 suddenly became the most beautiful number in the whole world to me.

I glanced over at Matt, and he looked overjoyed, too. In fact, for the first time in 24+ years of marriage, I saw him do an eyeball twirl! A special skill Matt developed while in junior high, an "eyeball twirl" begins when a person looks straight up briefly with both eyes, and then turns both eyeballs together in a quick clockwise motion. We followed the nurse's orders and celebrated that wonderful moment quietly. The fact that Matt looked truly goofy provided an extra bonus.

At about 3:30 in the morning, before my prayer for a 93 could begin, the respiratory therapist came in and moved Elizabeth's oxygen support through the ventilator from 100 percent down to 95. We'd seen evidence of God at work.

Soon after, Matt and I were asked to leave Elizabeth's room so they could take another x-ray. We sat together in the quiet waiting room. I looked at my husband—amazed at how close I felt to him. We both love our Elizabeth immensely. Now, as we stared death in the face, our need for each other intensified.

We persevered with internal prayers for Elizabeth to make good progression on her saturation abilities. By early morning, they'd moved her ventilator oxygen support level down to 90 percent. After a while, the night ended, and the hospital's busy morning routine began.

When Maggie, Sarah, and John returned to the hospital waiting room that morning, we told them about the "beautiful number 92" and how God gradually helped Elizabeth to get down to the 90 percent oxygen support level.

"We could see her improve one small step at a time as we prayed," I said. "Then around 3:30, they adjusted her ventilator for the first time."

When I mentioned the time, John had an interesting look on his face.

"Really?" he asked. "I woke up suddenly around three o'clock. I was reminded of the night my grandpa died. I remembered the phone rang at three a.m. My mom came into my bedroom to tell me he had passed away."

"So last night, when I woke up, a really bad fear came over me," John continued. "I was afraid a phone call would come from the hospital with bad news about Elizabeth. So I started praying for her. Finally, my fear began to melt away—and no phone call came."

Then Sarah joined in. "I woke up like that, too!" she said. "It was about three-fifteen. My heart was pounding. I felt really nervous and short of breath. I just knew I had to pray for Elizabeth right then, so I did. I checked my alarm clock a little later and it was three-twenty-seven."

We found out God also sent a "wake up and pray" call at 3 a.m. to another friend in Camarillo. And in the hallway of Elizabeth's dorm back at Biola, her roommates and the entire second floor of her dorm were also awake. Huddled together to keep warm, they prayed fervently for their Almighty God to heal their beloved friend's desperately sick lungs!

Only God knows how many more believers He not-so-gently nudged awake in the very early hours of April 20, 2004 to pray for Elizabeth.

Matt and I were tired after being up all night, but we did our best to regroup for another day. Soon, a few other church friends arrived, anxious for an update. While we updated them, we saw Dr. Abergel go into radiology across the hall from ICU. We thought he'd get Elizabeth's latest x-ray results and we were eager to hear from him. We hoped for good news.

But as we updated our friends with the overnight report, we realized God had already been faithful to answer many prayers since the crisis began. The Holy Spirit prompted us to give thanks. Our small group scooted chairs close together so we could hold hands and pray. We started by praising God that Elizabeth had survived the night. We also thanked Him for the improving ventilator numbers. Then we asked God to continue healing her.

While we prayed, Dr. Abergel came to the waiting room to talk with us. I briefly looked up and saw him there. For a moment I thought we should stop to see what he had to tell us. Then I remembered who we were already talking to—Almighty God. I motioned to Dr. Abergel to let him know I saw him and then continued to pray with the others. With priorities straight, we finished our talk with the Great Physician and then met with Dr. Abergel to hear the latest update.

"First of all, Elizabeth is significantly better," he said. "Her ventilator oxygen levels are down to 85 percent from 100 percent." Dr. Abergel spoke with the kind and caring voice we'd begun to appreciate.

For a few moments, I felt encouraged. But I could tell by his serious expression he had more to say.

"Even though she's improved some, Elizabeth remains critical," he said. "It's still fifty-fifty. Her lungs and heart are still in danger. Our hope is that she'll move to at least 70 percent by the end of the day."

It was difficult to keep up with Dr. Abergel as he continued to update us on Elizabeth's condition.

"Her lungs continue to be tight—they show signs of fibrosis (scarring)," he added. "Her blood sugars are up, similar to type 2 diabetes. She also has excess air trapped at the sides of her lungs."

The list seemed to go on and on. "Elizabeth isn't nearly out of the woods yet," he said finally. "We'll know within the next twelve- to forty-eight hours whether she'll pull through this."

We'd noticed a frightening swelling of Elizabeth's body. Her face, neck, hands, arms, upper body—pretty much all of her—looked inflated like an inner tube. So we asked the doctor about it. He explained that her illness was causing her metabolism to shoot up which, in turn, made her malnourished. Normally a healthy body takes protein into the bloodstream, which holds on to water in the nourishment process. Her condition decreased the amount of protein in her blood, so there was nothing present to hang on to the water and cause it to be eliminated in the usual way. Fluids began to seep into her skin and lungs instead. The general swelling we saw was caused by these fluids. The doctor told us it was a normal reaction.

So, the concerns of "Day 1", the first day of crisis—and then some—spilled over to the next. We were told Elizabeth's condition could still change very quickly, and Dr. Abergel continued to prioritize all her problems based on whether they were life-threatening or not. Meanwhile, Elizabeth teetered between life and death. While we felt helpless, we didn't feel hopeless; God's Word reminded us that the good hand of our God was upon Elizabeth and all of us.

I'd brought a tote bag to carry the special items I'd begun to accumulate. Tami came to the waiting room to deliver more sheets of Bible verses to help us keep our focus fixed on Jesus. I put them in my bag. Then I reported Elizabeth's significant overnight ventilator improvements to her before she left.

"I love it! I love it!" Tami exclaimed, as her eyes lit up.

While we waited through the morning hours, we'd received no new information. Waiting without information manufactured new questions. Unanswered questions tortured us.

To say many people were praying for Elizabeth is an understatement! The first night of the crisis, representatives from eight churches and a Christian university had joined with us in fervent prayer for her. God mass-produced new prayer support everywhere those original prayer warriors went. Passionate prayer requests were sent to all known connections—Bible studies, prayer groups, and prayer chains in many places.

At Biola University, John gave prayer requests to his many contacts and Elizabeth's roommates began a ribbon campaign that spread all over campus reminding students and professors to pray for Elizabeth.

Jeri gave encouraging motivation to a group she'd asked to pray.

"God loves these odds. It's time to watch Him work."

Of course, every crisis demands getting accurate information, thinking, and decision-making. But God wanted to teach us what to think about and what not to think about—another helpful aspect that would keep us in His place of refuge. Long hours of waiting had already proved to us that we could only think about Elizabeth's illness for so long. While our bodies were inactive, our minds and spirits were open all day for input. Terrifying, negative thoughts continued to race in. The facts in Elizabeth's case were grim—slightly improved, but still grim. God wanted us to learn that after we'd handled everything that was necessary, we needed to stop thinking about it. God wanted us to shift our thoughts back to Him.

Shifting thoughts in that way required skill at taking our thoughts captive. It also took great self-control. Since we were by no means experts at serious thought control, the Lord had to train and enable us as we went through each day. Hour by hour, we realized we were safe and strong only as long as we looked to the Lord and believed, with all our might, in His words and His ability to help Elizabeth. That activity protected us from destruction. We knew no other way to make it through our ordeal.

As I sat in a temporarily empty waiting room for a few minutes that afternoon, I thought back to 17 years ago. Spring was the time of year when Elizabeth would start psyching up for summer water fun. When she was a little girl, we lived in hot summer climates. Playing in water was the way to cool off. Every day she could, she wanted to "swim."

Once I said "yes" to the pool idea for the day, Elizabeth would squeal with delight. For her to "swim", we needed to set up a small inflatable plastic pool. It meant blowing air into two or three rings which made up the sides of the pool.

Each time I began setting up the pool, she could hardly wait until it was ready. But she did have to wait. Filling even a little pool with water took time. For a child, it's an agonizingly slow time. However, her enthusiasm began to build after the hose was turned on and she could see water cover the bottom area of the pool. As it rose slowly one inch after another, a wide smile of anticipation covered Elizabeth's face. She knew the fun was about to begin.

"What I wouldn't give to switch the day we're having with one like that!" I thought.

⁂

Many people who'd begun to pray for Elizabeth on Day 1—and those who woke up and prayed in the early hours of the night—were eager for an update on her condition. Telephone calls ate up hours of the day. Boy, did we repeat ourselves! If I wasn't the one delivering the latest update "speech" on the phone, Matt would be doing it. Phone weariness produced its own brand of exhaustion.

Ventilator work proceeded slowly one 5 percent step at a time throughout the day. They moved Elizabeth to a lower level a few times, but she wasn't able to sustain it. So they'd move her back to the previous setting. Then they'd try again later. By midday, she was at 80 percent.

By afternoon, some Biola students who'd been at the hospital with us the previous night came back again, joined by other students who'd been unable to come earlier. While they were there, we had another prayer session. Again, all were welcomed to participate. These students and their committed, ministering hearts impressed us once more. It was easy to see they loved God and Elizabeth, and were serious about praying for a miracle.

Toward evening, a wise nurse took it upon herself to give us a reality speech.

"You need to go home and get some sleep," she said, knowing Matt and I had been up throughout the previous night with Elizabeth. "You can't keep up such an unrealistic pace. If you try, you could get sick yourselves. Then you won't be any good for Elizabeth."

She also told us to encourage Elizabeth's friends in the waiting room to get back to school and keep up with their studies.

"It would be wrong for them to let the hard work of most of a semester go now," she said.

We decided to take her advice. With a recent report that Elizabeth's ventilator setting had been moved down to the 70 percent mark and that she was doing well with that, I was able to send her friends back to school with good news. I thanked them for coming and asked them to keep praying.

Matt and I knew we needed to follow the nurse's advice as well, but I wasn't ready to go just yet. As I spent quiet time in Elizabeth's room before leaving that evening, my mind went back to a recent, awful, unresolved conflict Elizabeth and I had experienced.

It all started a couple of months earlier when Matt's mom decided to close out a joint bank account. She gave him the sum of money she'd inherited from her own mother. He decided to divide it four ways between us and each of our daughters to help a little with their private college tuitions.

We'd encouraged Elizabeth to work part time during college to help with expenses. She didn't always feel like doing it, but she did it anyway. That semester, though, Elizabeth had decided not to work. I knew her example was crucial to our two younger daughters, but she wasn't aware how much we'd always counted on it. We didn't talk about it much, but I could tell we'd begun to have differing viewpoints. However, our "work part-time during college" policy my husband and I had set in motion still seemed good to us. We felt we needed to insist that Elizabeth get a job. We didn't want to give her the gift if she wouldn't work. However, she was our firstborn and we were new at learning to "let go" as parents.

With a visit to Biola approaching, we looked forward to spending some time with Elizabeth. I knew I needed to talk about the touchy subject, and I tried to prepare myself. I loved spending time with her and didn't want a conflict.

I foolishly picked a terrible time to jump into it. As we walked together to a class I'd been looking forward to sitting in on with her, I tried to explain our feelings about the part-time job.

Just before we went inside, I delivered my bomb ultimatum: "You don't get the money from Grandma unless you get a part-time job." Perhaps I could have worded that a little more carefully, but I didn't.

Elizabeth seemed shocked by my harsh words. Her face showed more anger than I'd ever seen before. In fact, she'd rarely been angry with me in past years. "You really won't give me this gift unless I get a job?" she asked in disbelief.

"That's right," I responded simply.

Just then we entered her class and sat down, both of us feeling devastated that this blew up in our faces when it did. I didn't expect such a reaction from Elizabeth.

Her professor was a wonderful teacher, but neither of us enjoyed the class like we'd planned. My heart was broken. My daughter was so angry with me. We couldn't talk about it any more until her class was over. I didn't understand what was going on.

After class we sat down on a nearby grass field under a tree and talked. Elizabeth tried to explain her reasons for not wanting to work. She also described how much was going on in her life at that time. Her senior classes were very hard. She'd just started to date John, her first boyfriend. She told me she didn't know how to date and she felt a little nervous about it.

Elizabeth was also in the middle of trying to figure out what to do with her life. She felt a lot of pressure to apply for graduate schools, mostly from her dad and me. As she pursued that goal, she found tests were required in the application process, which just placed another demand on her overwhelming schedule. It was almost too much!

"Do I want to go to graduate school right after I graduate?" she wondered. "Or should I get a full time job? What do I really want to do?" She just wasn't sure at that point.

She couldn't see any scraps of time available for holding a job right then. She still had some money in the bank, and she'd already figured out how to live meagerly. Her main expense was gas for her car. She hardly did anything that cost money. And a lot of her friends weren't working that semester.

As she explained all of this, she said she felt like I didn't care. I didn't appear to understand or to even be trying to understand. Actually, I was still stuck on a picture of Elizabeth's extremely angry face in my mind. I did have a list of pressures of my own Elizabeth didn't know about since she hadn't been at home for a while.

We'd each independently made up our minds about the issue, but we hadn't spoken to each other about it. The situation was new to us. Elizabeth's growing independence was a good thing, but it would take us a while to get used to it.

There wasn't enough time to talk much more before we had to drive home. We didn't resolve our conflict that day, so I rode home from Biola with a heavy, unsettled heart. Elizabeth and I had never talked about that part-time job ultimatum since then.

"Now her life is in such jeopardy," I thought. "Why didn't I take the initiative to talk more about this and clear it up before now?"

Before I left the ICU that night, her respiratory therapist looked me straight in the eye and said, "We're going to do everything we can to help your daughter." His bold, verbal commitment on behalf of the hospital team bolstered us up.

As our own normal bedtime drew near, I had to admit it had been a long two days. The idea of sleep held great appeal. We took the nurse's advice for ourselves and went home. Our bodies finally told us how tired they were during the five-minute drive home. When we got there, though, the answering machine light blinked and reminded us we couldn't get away from the demand for information. Those who couldn't reach us at the hospital called and left messages at the house—17 in all!

"I'm so thankful so many people are praying for Elizabeth!" I said. "But, I'm clueless about how to handle this massive desire for information!"

At that moment, however, the only thing we could think about was our desperate need for rest. As for me—once I dropped into bed, I slept like a baby.

CHAPTER FIVE

Surrender

THE NEXT MORNING AT THE hospital, Elizabeth remained in bed in a drug-induced coma. She was beginning Day 3 since her crisis began—overall, her 9th day in the hospital. At home, we were also in bed, just waking up after a good night's rest. Matt and I both needed it more than we knew.

However, the joy of a refreshed morning was dampened by a horrible question that ran through our minds while we got ready—"What if Elizabeth dies today?" The question was too dreadful to verbalize. I think we all felt that question would hold less power over us if we kept it inside. We rushed through breakfast, showers, and getting dressed so we could get back to Elizabeth as soon as possible. I gathered up my purse and tote bag and whatever else I thought would come in handy for a long day at the hospital. Hurrying out the door, I grabbed a couple of cards that had come in the mail—still unopened—so I could read them later.

"I read some encouraging verses in my quiet time this morning," said Matt as he drove us to the hospital. "Would you like to read them?"

"Sure," I said.

He knew I'd been bringing my Bible with me each day so I had it handy. He told me the reference and I read the verses quietly.

> "Where can I go from your Spirit? Where can I flee from your presence? If I go up to the heavens, you are there; if

I make my bed in the depths, you are there. If I rise on the wings of the dawn, if I settle on the far side of the sea, even there your hand will guide me; your right hand will hold me fast. If I say, 'Surely the darkness will hide me and the light become night around me,' even the darkness will not be dark to you, the night will shine like the day, for darkness is as light to you" (Psalm 139:7–12).

"These are good verses!" I said.

"Yeah. They make me feel like I know God will lead me and His right hand will hold me, no matter what happens. Even in the darkness of Elizabeth's illness, His light will continue to shine through my life," said Matt.

"I love it when God takes the time to reassure us of His presence," I said. "He *is* good."

"I've also been noticing these past two days that the Holy Spirit has been comforting me in a new, powerful way," Matt went on. "That's been great!"

I couldn't believe my eyes and ears! God was using our family crisis and the new, unusually heavy demands that had been placed on Matt as the head of the home to deepen his faith even more. He was discovering that even with such demands, God's provision was bigger. Watching this was thrilling and incredible!

✺

Shortly after we arrived at the hospital that morning, we got an update from Dr. Abergel, which contained good news and bad news. Optimistic, even with the worst cases, he began his report—in typical fashion—with the good news.

"Everything is looking better," he said. "Elizabeth had a very good night. Her ventilator level is now at 65 percent, and we should be able to drop it down again."

Three concerns made up the bad news. First, the morphine and paralysis medications she was receiving were beginning to cause problems with her digestive system. They planned to insert a stomach tube to keep it from shutting down.

Second, her blood pressure was high, which may have been caused by the stress of her illness, improper sedation, or pain. I had assumed the paralysis medication stopped her pain, but it didn't. While under its influence, Elizabeth may have felt pain, but she would have been unable to tell anyone about it.

Last, her heart rate remained very high, which still concerned the doctor. He didn't mention a chance of survival percentage at that time.

"She's still critically ill, but she's moving in the right direction," he said, doing his best to sound hopeful again. He scanned her chart and added, "Elizabeth is what . . . twenty-two, right. She's young and strong. That's definitely in her favor."

Again we updated family and friends. Some stopped by the hospital, but many received updates from us by cell phone. People were always grateful for any new information.

I'd recently noticed God's working in Matt's life, but He had work to do in me as well. In the busyness of our situation, He spoke to my heart and asked me a tough question.

Are you willing to let Me take Elizabeth home?

His disturbing question crossed my mind so clearly. As He drew me in to consider it, He didn't say He would definitely take her home; He just asked if I was willing to let Him do so, if He chose to.

"Lord, I can't think about this," I responded at first. "I don't want to think about this. And there isn't time to think about this. There are so many things on my mind as it is. I'm here in a busy hospital, with visitors in and out throughout the day. I just can't think about such a serious question, Lord.

Make time to think about it, God said.

He pushed me to face that very real possibility. He wouldn't let me off the hook. He waited for me to ponder His heart-rending question.

"As a parent, this is the worst thing you could ask of me," I told God. "Lord, please don't ask this! I want Elizabeth to stay here. For me to let my child die goes against what it means to be a parent. I don't know how to do it. I just want her to be okay."

When I mentioned God's question to Matt, he said God had asked him the same thing. He'd been silently thinking it through himself. At first he didn't know how to respond to God.

"Lord, I'm not sure I'll be able to keep trusting you if you take Elizabeth home," Matt told God. "What if it decreases my faith?"

"I know there's a chance Elizabeth may die and I'm afraid of her dying," Matt thought. "I don't want that to happen. I don't want to be a parent who lost a child. I want to die first—before my children. Besides, she's a big part of our family and it would leave a big hole if she died."

While we both thought over this horrible question God had put before us, we each felt a little like Abraham when God told him to sacrifice Isaac.

> "Then God said, 'Take your son, your only son, Isaac, whom you love, and go to the region of Moriah. Sacrifice him there as a burnt offering on one of the mountains I will tell you about'" (Genesis 22:2).

Elizabeth was not our only daughter, but she was our only *Elizabeth*. There was no one like her. However, we wanted to be strong in faith and willing to act on whatever God told us to do.

"Am I willing, like Abraham?" I had to ask myself.

"Lord, help me be willing," I prayed.

We remembered how carefully God watched Abraham.

> "Now I know that you fear God, because you have not withheld from me your son, your only son" (Genesis 22:12).

We knew how that story ended—God spared Isaac's life and richly blessed Abraham afterward.

When God posed His question to me, He promised no specific outcome. He didn't tell me He'd spare her life as He did Isaac's. He was fixed on attaining our unconditional surrender. He kept waiting for the answer to His question. I could feel His gaze upon me.

When we weren't allowed in Elizabeth's room for an unusually long period of time that day, we wondered if other problems had developed. When I went in for a mid-morning visit with Elizabeth, Dr. Abergel walked toward me. His expression was serious and I had to ask him how Elizabeth was doing.

"She only has a 40 percent chance of survival now," Dr. Abergel said.

This was actually worse than the 50 percent prognosis from the previous day.

Then the doctor gestured with his thumb and forefinger barely an inch apart and said, "I'll give her about this much hope."

"We'll take it," I said.

I felt a tiny amount of hope was better than no hope. After he left, I walked to the cabinet and started to put on my isolation garb.

From day to day, the Lord had revealed the path to His place of refuge during our calamity. His commitment to do this for His people is explained by Isaiah.

> "I will lead the blind by ways they have not known, along unfamiliar paths I will guide them; I will turn the darkness into light before them and make the rough places smooth. These things I will do. I will not forsake them" (Isaiah 42:16).

There was no way God was smoothing our path before us because we were just a nice family with a good attitude. We were simply in the hands of God and He was at work. This smoothness was such an unbelievable discovery to us.

Meanwhile, John found it difficult to know what to do each day. He'd returned to Biola the previous night to attempt normal college life again. But not long after morning began, he wasn't sure he should be there.

"What am I doing here?!" he asked himself. "It's so strange to sit around a hospital all day and wonder if my girlfriend will make it. But here at school, no one can answer my constant question: 'How is Elizabeth?' I can't stop thinking about her!"

He realized he belonged back at the hospital, so he made plans to return as soon as he could.

That afternoon Maggie and Sarah prepared to see their sister again. They hadn't visited in her room for two days. It had been difficult for them that first day to see her unconscious and hooked up to all kinds of medical equipment. Sarah had seen her briefly one other time through the glass door of her room. She told us Elizabeth's eyes were partly open, but they didn't register anything. That scared Sarah and left her hesitant to visit. Maggie, too, felt uneasy.

Before the girls went in, Matt and I told them Elizabeth would look even less like herself, since her body was much more swollen from the excess fluids seeping into her skin.

As Sarah prepared for her visit, she thought hard about what to say. She'd heard Elizabeth's blood pressure numbers meant she could possibly be in a lot of pain. Her high heart rate could have been caused, in part, by anxiety about what was happening to her. Sarah tried to find words that would ease Elizabeth's mind.

We decided that the girls would come with me one at a time. Maggie came first. As we entered, we received a kind reminder from Elizabeth's nurse.

"It's calming and encouraging for her to have you in her room—she's able to hear you and knows you're there, even though she isn't conscious."

So, as Maggie held one of Elizabeth's hot, puffy hands, she did her best to carry on a one-sided conversation. I noticed she hesitated to look toward her sister's un-Elizabeth-like face as she talked.

After a brief visit, Maggie and Sarah switched places. The nurse gave Sarah the same reminder. Sarah also nervously avoided a direct look at Elizabeth's face. In her one-sided conversation, she shared her cheerful thoughts with Elizabeth, telling her to think of God as her pain medication. Then she went on to talk about happy memories we'd shared as a family.

As they ended their visits, each sister sweetly told Elizabeth how much she loved her. Then we noticed Elizabeth's high heart rate had calmed down a little. Maggie and Sarah's presence and conversation appeared to make a difference to Elizabeth. I was proud to see them face their fear and spend important time with their big sister.

That day the Lord provided clear thinking time for Matt and me about His question. He gradually worked in our hearts and made it possible for us to desire His will.

He'd guided me to a place I never thought I'd find myself.

When I was ready, I gave God my answer. I stood alone in the hospital restroom—of all places—and closed the door on the outside world. In the momentary quietness of my unusual little "prayer chapel," I whispered my answer to my God.

"Yes, Lord, I'm willing for You to take Elizabeth, if that's Your plan for her life. It's up to you . . . I won't stand in Your way. But I can't dwell on this possibility for too long. Lord, I will continue to ask You to heal Elizabeth."

Throughout the day, God had reassured Matt He would help him walk in faith like Abraham, whatever the outcome. He came to believe his faith would not be shaken if the Lord took Elizabeth home. Individually, we both gave God the same answer. We surrendered our daughter's life to the sovereign choice of God.

Because this surrender process had gone on in my heart, I began to mention the possibility to people around me that Elizabeth may not survive. Most people seemed bothered by it, and whether they conveyed it out loud or not, their reactions seemed to say: "Don't you believe God can do the impossible?"

"Yes, I do believe!" I thought. "I know He can heal my daughter."

But by that time, I'd become totally aware that God might choose to answer our prayers with a "no." Either way, we were determined to trust Him—whether Elizabeth's reports were good or bad. From then on, Matt and I decided to keep our surrender experiences to ourselves.

God faithfully provided fresh encouragement through those who stopped by. One friend returned to the waiting room later that afternoon with a big white envelope full of pages of Bible verses and inspirational notes she'd copied for us which perfectly addressed our need. After reading some of them, we put them with Tami's in my ever-present tote bag so we could refer to them often.

That's when I noticed the unopened cards I'd brought from home that morning. I decided it was a good time to read them. The first one I opened reminded me of yet another way God was providing help. Romans 8:34 tells us that Jesus is at the right hand of God (the position of power), interceding for us.

Hebrews 7:25 also says Jesus "always lives to intercede for them" (those who come to God through Him).

So Jesus was the glorious prayer warrior at the head of the team of believers committed to pray for Elizabeth and our family. I'd forgotten that awesome, ongoing ministry of Jesus.

I took a few minutes to think about what "intercede" means. A person who intercedes speaks and pleads for another. He may possibly ask a favor or offer reasons and excuses for them. Pleading in prayer may become so earnest, it leads to begging.

In the Old Testament, we find the story of a man longing for an intercessor, a role perfectly fulfilled only by Jesus Christ in New Testament times. This man is Job. He was a blameless, upright man of faith experiencing intense suffering. False accusations from his friends added to his deep agony.

Somehow, while going through emotional cycles of grief, Job occasionally had moments when extraordinary hope burst through. He caught a glimpse of his only hope—a heavenly intercessor who would plead with God on his behalf.

> "Even now, behold, my witness is in heaven and my advocate is on high. My friends are my scoffers; my eye weeps to God. O that a man might plead with God as a man with his neighbor!" (Job 16:19–21 NASB).

I tried to wrap my mind around this—Jesus was appearing in the Father's presence for us. I wondered what He was actually praying about during our crisis. I remembered His prayer for believers recorded in John 17. In those verses, He prayed for believers on a deeply spiritual level to have such things as protection from evil, unity with God and one another, holiness, and the full measure of His love, joy, and presence. He also prayed for His followers to see His glory. There was no way for us to know exactly how Jesus was interceding for us in our circumstances, but I was sure He was praying for our deepest needs. We may not have been aware of them, but He alone saw them clearly.

As I continued thinking about Jesus' intercessory prayers, verses about the Holy Spirit's praying also came to mind.

> "In the same way, the Spirit helps us in our weakness. We do not know what we ought to pray for, but the Spirit Himself intercedes for us with groans that words cannot express. And He who searches our hearts knows the mind of the Spirit, because the Spirit intercedes for the saints in accordance with God's will" (Romans 8:26–27).

I was so encouraged when I thought of such passionate assistance from God even at that very moment. Elizabeth's need was God-sized and the Father provided God-sized help through the Son and the Holy Spirit. Almighty, holy power was at work—the greatest source of power in the universe! In our helpless state, we were fully backed up by God Himself. It was thrilling to ponder those awesome facts! We were truly blessed!

The second card came from Jeri. In it she included a copy of a poem she'd written when she went through her own near-death experience years ago.

The Moment of Inbetween

In the moment of inbetween I found You.
Inbetween sleep and awake, life and death, You are there
Not a bright light beckoning or coaxing,
But a gentle presence
Calming, soothing, casting out fear;
For who can fear love?
In joyous communion
You heard my heart's feeble songs of praise
Without pretense.
And believing my spirit's true confession,

You relinquished me to life
In that fragile, Holy moment of inbetween.
By Jeri Chrysong
Feb. 12, 1993

Even though I'd come to a place of acceptance about the possibility that Elizabeth might not make it, I kept doing my best not to think about it much. But after dinner that evening, as Matt and I prepared to return to ICU, we received a cruel reminder. When Matt reached for the ICU door handle, the door suddenly swung open.

We moved out of the way while two hospital transport employees wheeled out a gurney carrying a patient who'd recently died. A sheet covered the head. I quickly turned away and stepped into the nearby prayer chapel. A quick chill of fear shivered through my heart. The scene was too close for comfort.

CHAPTER SIX

Spiritual Roller Coaster

MATT AND I DECIDED THAT night to stay in Elizabeth's room in shifts. I'd stay until about 2:30 a.m. while he went home to sleep. Then we'd switch places. Thoughts of ongoing heavenly intercession buoyed me up and filled me with God's peace as I walked into my daughter's room and sat down at her bedside.

"What do you want me to do while I'm here with Elizabeth?" I asked the Lord.

Diane, sing to Me again, He whispered.

We'd already sung in her room on the first critical night. I hadn't given singing much thought since then. Somehow, it seemed a little easier to sing with the majority of a worship band present.

Remember how much you and Elizabeth both love worshipping Me whenever you get a chance? God asked. *Just start. It will be good.*

So I yielded to the Holy Spirit's control.

Before I started, I asked Elizabeth's nurse if it would be okay if I sang.

"It will be fine as long as her heart and blood pressure rates don't increase," she said. "Don't forget she's an extremely fragile young woman."

Then she left the room. After I quieted my heart, I began to sing an old favorite which starts out: "His name is wonderful. His name is wonderful. His name is wonderful, Jesus my Lord . . ."

At first, I kept my eye on the monitor and numbers. They seemed to stay steady, so I continued to sing any chorus or hymn God brought to mind. In no time, I really started to enjoy it. I found myself thinking less about my daughter's illness and more about my God who held her in His hands. The longer I sang, the clearer my focus became on the Lord.

A little later the nurse came back into Elizabeth's room to check her IV. I asked her if she knew any praise and worship songs. She told me she and her son really liked "Swing Low, Sweet Chariot." Suddenly, her clear, lovely voice filled the room.

> "Swing low, sweet chariot,
> Comin' for to carry me home.
> Swing low, sweet chariot,
> Comin' for to carry me home."[5]

"Oh, this is so beautiful!" I thought. "I can't believe I'm hearing such a delightful voice singing about God in Elizabeth's ICU room!"

However, I don't think she considered what the words of "Swing Low, Sweet Chariot" suggested. When I heard the phrase "comin' for to carry me home," I felt uneasy. I really didn't want God's chariot to come carry Elizabeth home to heaven just yet. After the nurse left, I attempted to fix my dilemma with the phrase.

"Elizabeth, won't it be exciting when God comes back to take all His people home to heaven . . . in the future?" I said, leaning toward her.

"Time for a different song," I thought. "Let's see, the nurse also suggested 'In the Garden.' How does the first verse go? Oh yeah. 'I come to the garden alone . . .'"

The chorus was especially good. When I sang it, my heart thrilled at the profound truth there—"He tells me I am His own." The words were so good, I sang them again.

> "And He walks with me, and He talks with me,
> And He tells me I am His own;

---

5   "Swing Low, Sweet Chariot" Traditional Spiritual. Public domain.

> And the joy we share as we tarry there, none other has
> ever known."[6]

As I continued singing bold words that spoke of His great love, the Holy Spirit kept working in my heart, weeding out all thoughts about anything or anyone but God. My focus on Him became sharper. The words I sang became more real than ever. It was as if they woke up and sprang to new life in me.

When I took a break, I was surprised to feel so overwhelmed by joy. This joy followed me out of Elizabeth's room and down the hall, and gave me extra energy!

During my break, I realized my repertoire of songs was running low.

"Lord, I need more ideas of songs to sing," I said.

He floated the chorus which starts out "The joy of the Lord is my strength . . ." across my mind.

"That explains what I'm feeling right now, Lord—Your joy!" I exclaimed. "And I can't believe how strong it's making me feel!"

I immediately began to sing that song quietly.

As I walked back to her room, the Lord's joy mounted within me more and more by the minute. I snapped my fingers and hummed "the joy of the Lord is my strength" a couple more times. I couldn't wait to sing again "with" Elizabeth. Once back in her room, I checked the numbers on the monitor. They still looked fine.

The Lord quickly prepared my heart for more worship. Elizabeth remained still and asleep. I closed my eyes and sat calmly for a few minutes. Then I began to sing.

The Lord prompted song after song. While I sang, the heavenly focus God gave me became complete. It felt like no one else was in the world except God, Elizabeth, and me. Between songs, a holy stillness filled her room. It felt like time stood still.

"Something powerful is going on here!" I thought.

While I tried to comprehend it, the Lord brought a Scripture verse to my mind.

"Yet You are holy, O You who are enthroned upon the praises of Israel" (Psalm 22:3 NASB.)

---

[6] "In the Garden." Words and music by C. Austin Miles. Public domain.

I took that to mean God was also enthroned upon *my* praises. As I sang, I'd placed God in the highest place of authority over our lives. The sovereign Lord sat on His throne in that ICU room. He'd been right there with us all along, and I believed, again, that Elizabeth worshipped along with me in spirit. I'd been experiencing the deepest, most focused worship of my life!

But I still couldn't help wondering about one thing.

"How can God bless me so richly while my daughter's life lingers "inbetween" life and death?" I thought.

I sat quietly in the Lord's presence a little longer.

The next song idea to come to me was, "The Easter Song"—a cherished family song that we usually sing at home on Easter Sunday morning. Elizabeth was unable to sing it that year since she was sick. The song begins softly, but I'd forgotten that it gets much louder and high-pitched at the end. I'd also forgotten to look at her monitor for quite a while. I just kept singing. With each word, my excitement and volume built. I continued singing, unaware that the loud, exciting end of the song was over-stimulating Elizabeth.

The nurse came in and told me Elizabeth's numbers were rising and I had to leave. A little sadness and fear mixed with my abundant joy.

"What if I caused Elizabeth harm?" I asked the nurse.

"She will calm down after you leave," she said. "She probably needed this encouragement about now."

Her kind words as I got ready to leave the hospital earlier than I'd planned prevented me from feeling too terrible about making Elizabeth's numbers rise.

Since the nurse felt it may be better to let Elizabeth have some quiet rest through the night, she recommended I have Matt call the ICU before he came in at 3:00 a.m. She also thought they might have to cancel his visit. If they cancelled, I knew he'd miss spending that time with her.

While I drove home close to midnight, I thought I might burst with joy and excitement over the worship and praise "concert" I'd just given Elizabeth. I thought to myself how much I would have missed if I hadn't followed God's earlier prompting to sing.

When I got home, I was disappointed to find the house completely dark. Everyone had already gone to bed. But I felt like I just had to tell someone about what had happened. Maggie ordinarily loves to stay up late, so I was shocked to see her light out so early. I gently knocked on her door and went inside.

"Maggie? Are you awake?" I whispered.

No answer. I moved closer to her bed and whispered again. I couldn't help it; I had to tell someone what happened!

She gave a faint whisper and moved a little. I took this as a sign that God had given me someone to listen to my story. So I sat on the edge of Maggie's bed in the dark and told her all about my unbelievable, joy-filled evening of song. She seemed to enjoy the story, and I felt so much better letting my joy overflow.

I left her room so she could go back to sleep. Then I wrote a note for Matt.

"I over-stimulated Elizabeth, so the nurse said to call her before you go in."

I got ready for bed quickly, still overjoyed. Soon I'd joined the house full of sleeping family members. None of us were aware how much we needed the restoring power of sleep in order to meet the challenges of the day ahead.

By the next morning, Elizabeth had been in ICU for seven days. We'd trusted Dr. Abergel with her medical care for over three of those days, since her condition became life-threatening. He continued to work tirelessly—late into the night, every night. Always open to new treatments and suggestions from colleagues, he searched to find anything able to help Elizabeth. He was devoted to her.

Actually we'd heard many glowing reports about Dr. Abergel as we spent hour upon hour at the hospital. One nurse felt he was the kind of doctor you want on your side in a time of crisis. An ER doctor shared his desire to have Dr. Abergel take care of him if he ever got into the same trouble as Elizabeth. He said Dr. Abergel was excellent.

It's one thing when other patients or families compliment their doctors, but when other doctors and nurses praise the physicians they work alongside, it means a lot. We easily fell in line with the crowd of Abergel admirers, but not only because many others highly respected him. We'd seen him in action ourselves and we already felt an incredible bond with Elizabeth's brilliant, exceptional doctor. Matt and I truly believed God picked him to provide his wonderful care for our daughter.

As he updated us that morning, Dr. Abergel changed her prognosis from the 40% chance of survival he'd predicted the day before, back to a 50/50 chance. At first, it sounded like she may have improved a little, but then he told us some problems had intensified. Her heart rate was still too high, and she needed medication to lower it. He was also concerned that she still needed paralysis medication. She'd used it for over three days and even so, the pressure in her lungs remained high. He knew prolonged use of the paralysis medication could lead to myopathy, a disease of the muscles. If that developed, it would slow her recovery or have long-range effects.

Elizabeth wasn't ready for visitors yet that morning, so we returned to the waiting room. I sat down under a landscape picture of birch trees and a lake that hung on the wall. Its subdued pink and blue colors caught my eye and attempted to soothe me.

As three days in intense prayer mode turned to four, I began to sense—I'd never prayed so much in my life! And God Himself continued to raise up believers devoted to praying for Elizabeth from a variety of places. All that prayer support really made me think. I don't believe He answers prayer only if large numbers of people pray. I do believe, in His wisdom, He answers every prayer offered in faith, even if there's only one prayer warrior alone who has His ear in a particular situation.

So why did He continue to enlist more people to pray so passionately and unceasingly for Elizabeth? It was a wonderful mystery. He orchestrated the prayer team and continuously prompted it to pray. Whatever His reasons, we stood in awe as we watched Him work through His faithful people. That prayer ministry was so far beyond us and our comprehension.

We sat in the waiting room the rest of the morning with no news. As morning turned to afternoon, we still weren't allowed in Elizabeth's room. We continued to wait and wonder a lot. I began to have a suffocating, sinking feeling. We checked again later and they finally gave us permission to see her for a brief time.

Before we entered her room, her nurse gave us instructions.

"Speak gently to Elizabeth and remain calm. Reassure her there are a lot of people looking out for her. And don't touch her."

It was clear from her words and demeanor that Elizabeth required even more delicate treatment now. Once inside, we noticed her appearance had changed since the day before. Her face and neck, red with fever, were quite a bit larger. Even the balls of her eyes appeared swollen. They looked golf-ball-sized with her eyelids stretched tightly over them.

"She looks so very sick! Would God take her home now?" I wondered.

By mid-afternoon, we were alone again in the waiting room with our thoughts. The uncertainty we'd experienced earlier in the day deepened. Matt and I felt a heaviness, a sense of danger and dread. Our requests to see Elizabeth again later were denied, which didn't help.

Elizabeth continued to worsen. Her body had become overwhelmed by the viral infection, and she wasn't responding to treatments. Somewhere behind those big blue ICU doors that kept us on the outside, Dr. Abergel talked to colleagues and decided what to do next to get Elizabeth through more tough hours. He knew she had absolutely no reserves at that point. Then, at around 4:00 that afternoon, we were called in.

The news wasn't good. Elizabeth had developed septic shock, also called sepsis. The doctor explained it was an overwhelming bacterial infection that invaded the entire body via the bloodstream. In addition, her heart rate had gone even higher while her blood pressure had gone lower, she'd developed a high fever, and her saturation levels had gotten worse, which was a setback. They'd been forced to increase her oxygen support level.

Dr. Abergel ended his update with haunting words: "We took a *big* step backwards!"

Matt and I both found the doctor's words disheartening.

Years before that day began, I'd secretly hoped my "whatever it takes" plea would mean I'd face a period of difficulty that would be pretty tough, but which I could handle. It turned out to be beyond my expectations, way beyond. In our calamity, we realized we needed God's help just to survive His work in our lives. The words "we took a big step backwards" made me feel like His gaze was directly upon me—and it was intense. At times, I longed for Him to look away again.

Now Elizabeth required new aggressive action. More blood tests were ordered, since the doctors wanted to make sure they hadn't missed anything. The infectious disease doctor had Elizabeth put on a cooling blanket, which circulated cool water under her body, and ice packs placed under her arms and in various other places to bring her fever down.

The doctor explained her sepsis problem briefly. He told us that, in order for blood to flow properly to vital organs, the blood vessels need to both dilate and constrict. However, toxins in Elizabeth's blood inhibited her blood vessels from constricting, causing her blood pressure to become low. Then the low blood pressure brought serious threats of injury to her vital organs—kidney failure, heart attack, or stroke.

That afternoon, Dr. Abergel had consulted an interventional cardiologist who suggested inserting a special catheter that could allow them to tightly control the amount of fluid they gave Elizabeth and bring it back into balance. They would insert the catheter into a vein and then thread it into her heart and pulmonary artery—the part of the heart that carries blood to and from the lungs. Dr. Abergel wanted the procedure done, but he needed our consent.

We realized Elizabeth's vital signs all reflected her poor condition. She continued to deteriorate. Even her nutritional status steadily worsened. It seemed like they were doing everything they could think of, yet improvement eluded her. We felt we had no choice, so we signed the consent form and returned to the waiting room.

In the early evening hours, we remained alone in the waiting room and the uneasiness gradually turned to intense fear. We hadn't heard anything in over two hours.

"Elizabeth's life could end while I sit here in this chair this very moment, or in ten minutes, or in half an hour," I thought. "Oh, Lord, what's going to happen to her?"

We felt as desperate and confused as we had on the first day of our crisis. By then, we felt the enormous burden for Elizabeth was too weighty for us to carry alone, and we knew she needed more prayer. So I called one of our church elders.

"Come and pray with us!" I requested urgently.

Then I asked him to invite anyone from church who was available to come. The Lord began compelling people to come. In no time, the waiting room was filled with precious believers. One man said he'd had his phones turned off, but one rang anyway to notify him to come pray again! We were so touched by those who were unafraid to draw near to us in our time of great need. The man with "God's phone service" definitely saw it as a priority.

Matt gave a brief update to the group and explained the new threat. Again, believers lifted their voices in prayer to our powerful, loving God.

"Thank You, Lord, for keeping Elizabeth alive through four critical days and nights. We praise You for that miracle."

Thank You for Your power and wisdom."

"Lord, we ask You to heal her from septic shock and from the lung infection."

"Please guide the hands of the doctor as he does the procedure."

"You know how much we want You to heal Elizabeth, but we leave that sovereign choice to You."

"We praise You for Your infinite capabilities."

"We praise You for all You will do."

"We put Elizabeth in Your hands."

"Thank You for Your presence with us and for hearing our prayers in Jesus' name."

We knew that the faith and support of God's praying people were ministering to Elizabeth's body, and it bolstered us up again.

Just as our prayer session ended, Elizabeth's ICU nurse came into the room.

"I don't know what you people have been doing in here, but keep it up!" she said. "There is no reason the procedure just went as well as it did."

We were amazed! We didn't know it, but we'd been in prayer at the very same time the procedure was taking place. We prayed, and God answered immediately.

A short time later, Dr. Abergel came into the waiting room to tell us that the new catheter's readings showed that Elizabeth's condition had already started to improve! We felt the burden lift. Intense joy and gratitude filled our hearts.

God performed another miracle that night. Death tried to snatch Elizabeth away again, but God drew her back into the land of the living.

CHAPTER SEVEN

Perfect, Faithful Provision

MATT'S A SCIENTIST WHO LOVES facts, so his mind thirsted for more information about septic shock. The medical staff hadn't seemed too concerned about it and appeared confident they'd take care of the problem. But in our hearts and spirits, we'd sensed her situation held a greater threat than they'd let on.

Before we left for the hospital the following morning, Matt hurried to the oak bookcase in our living room, slid the glass front upward, and pulled out our well-worn home medical guide. What he read told him more than he wanted to know: Shock, overwhelming infection, organ failure…death.

Realizing he'd heard similar phrases from the doctor, those words loitered uncomfortably in his mind. He chose to keep me uninformed about the facts he discovered and gave me only a general summary.

"Septic shock is much worse than they led us to believe. You don't want to know what I read," he said.

Every day we were painfully aware of how much we didn't understand. Before he pushed those fear-packed words from his mind, Matt had a question for me.

"How is an incredibly sick person supposed to get better when their blood is poisoned?" he asked.

"I have no idea," I said.

Our Ever-Present Help

In the waiting room that morning, we found evidence that Tami had already come and gone, leaving behind words of hope for us.

> "The Lord will guide you always; He will satisfy your needs in a sun-scorched land and will strengthen your frame. You will be like a well-watered garden, like a spring whose waters never fail" (Isaiah 58:11).

Our hospital day started with perfect promises from a perfect God.

We greeted Dr. Abergel at the ICU desk, and he began his update on Elizabeth. Despite a rocky night, things were "significantly better" that morning. Her heart rate and blood pressure were better, and so were her blood saturation and oxygen levels.

Since she looked so much better, Dr. Abergel wanted to repair one of the non-life-threatening problems that had been shelved earlier. Her lower left lung had been collapsed for days. Inserting a small pigtail chest tube in it could expand the lung properly again and give her another 20 percent lung capacity. He placed her on the radiologist's schedule to have the procedure done.

It was over quickly. The radiologist was smiling when he returned with his report.

"The procedure went very well," he said. "The excess air was released and the lung fully re-expanded."

Whenever "lung fully re-expanded" was pronounced in ICU, the medical staff smiled. It meant a chest tube procedure was successful. Before the procedure, Elizabeth's saturation level was 88, 89. Afterward, it went up to a 92.

When Elizabeth's crisis began, we were told about two critical oxygen support percentage goals. The first one was 70 percent, which she'd reached earlier in the week. The next milestone of 50 percent still loomed before us. We'd prayed intensely for her to reach that mark, but she was unable to do so. We wondered aloud what would happen since Elizabeth wasn't yet at the 50 percent level of ventilator support. Would this cause her serious problems?

"We'd all be thrilled if she'd been able to get to 50 percent, but she can't yet," Dr. Abergel replied.

He told us the head of respiratory therapy had devoted herself to solving the mystery of how to make ventilator progress with Elizabeth, since the conventional ways weren't working for her. After some trial and error, the respiratory therapist devised a method with new boundaries to get Elizabeth to lower ventilator levels and still keep her comfortable. This new method alleviated Dr. Abergel's earlier concern about reaching the 50 percent mark quickly.

We noticed the medical personnel working on Elizabeth's case shared a dedicated mindset. They racked their brains to discover anything that could help her. Many said they took Elizabeth home with them when they left work. One nurse said she was a patient you couldn't forget at the end of the day. She came to their minds when they woke up. Since Elizabeth was so young, they didn't want to lose her. Even Dr. Abergel felt that way.

"I fall asleep at night trying to figure out what else to do to help her," he said.

We prayed for the God of infinite wisdom to give them the understanding they so desperately desired.

Just one day earlier, no news had felt ominous. But that day, it felt like things were a little better. "No news was good news."

By late afternoon, our kids, John, and other friends began to urge Matt and me to take a break. They knew we'd been at the hospital all week except when we ate and slept. Maybe we looked worse than we realized. Eventually, they convinced both of us to go out.

We planned to see a movie. When it was time to go, we found neither of us knew how to actually walk away from the situation. We got our bodies out of the hospital building, but our hearts and minds stayed with our daughter in the hospital bed. When we sat down in the darkened theater, we slowly exhaled and tried to relax. I rocked back and forth a little in my theater seat. It felt good, but strange, to be out of the hospital.

However, it was a struggle to keep our minds on the rather dull movie we picked. We were glad when it ended. We felt like young parents who'd left their new baby with a babysitter for the first time. We hurried back to check on Elizabeth.

A small crowd had gathered in the waiting room while we were gone. It included Maggie, Sarah, John, Mary (Elizabeth's friend), Jeri and her son, Sam. As we approached the waiting room, we heard their pleasant conversations.

We checked in with Dr. Abergel at the ICU desk right away.

"How's Elizabeth?" Matt asked.

"She's continuing to move in the right direction, which is good," said Dr. Abergel.

By that time, I loved that phrase! I thought it was one of Dr. Abergel's favorites.

Then he began to list off many improvements that were shockingly good! While he talked, I started to notice he had teeth. During the previous long week, I didn't remember a time when I'd seen them, because I don't think he smiled all through the week. From Day 1 on, he'd only had grim, serious news to report. But that night, he smiled. It was hard to believe that within less than 24 hours of her septic shock danger, we were hearing almost an opposite report.

I told him I was sure he'd really like Elizabeth when she woke up. He said he already liked her a lot. He told us about their brief talk five days earlier, when they first took extreme measures to help her. He said he'd explained what they needed to do and she looked directly at him.

"Thank you for helping me," she said.

That meant a lot to him.

Dr. Abergel was about finished giving us the update.

"I'm going to move her up to a 70 percent chance of survival," he said.

Instantly I was intensely thrilled!

"This is huge!" I thought. "I can't contain this joy! I have to tell everyone!"

I smiled back at the doctor and then quickly headed for the door. My quick walk turned into a run. When I exited the door and turned toward the waiting room, I noticed Sam and John down the hall. As I ran toward them, I began to leap and jump for joy with all my might.

Their eyes bugged out and their mouths dropped open. After all, it's not every day people see a 52-year-old woman running and jumping toward them down a hospital hallway! I didn't know it, but Matt had followed me to the waiting room. We quickly passed on Dr. Abergel's report of a 70 percent chance of survival. Everyone erupted with excitement.

Our joy was humongous! We smiled. We cheered. We hugged. We exclaimed disbelief and wonder! We laughed. It was amazing! We made up for an almost smileless week ourselves that night. Jeri had her camera with her and she captured our reactions on film.

For as long as I've known him, Matt's had the same favorite Bible verse.

> "Do not be anxious about anything, but in everything, by prayer and petition, with thanksgiving, present your requests to God. And the peace of God, which transcends all understanding, will guard your hearts and your minds in Christ Jesus" (Philippians 4:6–7).

For five days, the words of these verses became Matt's way of life. He'd prayed about everything and God had exchanged his anxiety for peace. His faith was growing. A deeper rejoicing took place between us that night—rejoicing in the Lord.

Over the past five days, I'd discovered a new type of vision in God's place of refuge. I felt so close to the Lord there that I could see Him at work on Elizabeth's behalf. Since her first critical day, I'd had a front row seat to watch God exert His extraordinary force and divine power (the same power He used to resurrect Jesus) to begin her healing. His power is awesome! When it seemed her body couldn't improve, His power made the impossible possible. He'd supernaturally reversed the natural course of events. I'd seen incredible miracles!

While we celebrated in the waiting room, I got the feeling we were probably incredibly loud. At about 10:30 p.m., I suggested we move our joy to our house.

When we got home, we played the messages back off our packed answering machine. Clyde Cook, the president of Biola University at that time had left the final message. He told us he'd been out of the country at a conference and he'd just heard about Elizabeth. He assured us of his prayers for her and our family. Then he actually began praying over the phone for her. He lifted Elizabeth up before the Father, acknowledging that she belonged to Him and that His Spirit indwelt her, which made her body His temple.

"Father, repair Your temple and bring her back to full strength and health," he prayed. "Encourage and bless all her friends and loved ones. And thank you that you stand alongside of us in times like these."

Since we didn't know him personally, we were very impressed that he took the time to call our home and show his love and concern. We knew, as president of a growing Christian university, he had many responsibilities. We felt that in 95% of colleges, a call like his wouldn't have been made. But he took time to function like a caring shepherd overseeing one of his sheep in danger. He was tender and supportive.

The first time I saw Clyde, I was a student at Biola myself. It was close to thirty years earlier and he actually substituted once in one of my classes. He was a missions professor at that time. While I was busy getting married and raising my family, he'd become the president of Biola. The next time I saw him was when our family left Elizabeth there to begin her first semester. He was a humble, genuine man of God with a bold faith. He lived what he believed. If he said he'd pray for you, you knew he'd really do it. I was grateful for the influence he'd have on Elizabeth as a student. I admired him from afar whenever I visited Biola.

When he assured us of his prayer support for Elizabeth in his message, I felt like the Lord brought in a giant of the faith to help. He was a mature, seasoned believer experienced in standing strong through trials. It was encouraging in his message to hear him say *"we're* praying for Elizabeth and your family" because I knew that also meant the Biola community was praying—staff and students alike.

After listening to Clyde's message, our loud, celebrative mood resumed. A friend had delivered an exquisite dessert earlier and we ate that together. It added to our celebration.

"Who knew we'd have great news to celebrate that night?" I thought.

None of us realized how loud we were. But our neighbors did. Close to midnight, as Jeri and Sam were leaving, we went outside to say goodbye. We met a neighbor walking down the sidewalk toward our house. He was coming to find out what was causing all that racket.

"Elizabeth is still alive!" reverberated in hearts and minds all around the ICU the next morning. A rejoicing atmosphere permeated the place.

Witnessing miracles with their own two eyes absolutely astonished everyone involved!

Not long after we arrived at the hospital, I crossed paths in the hallway with an ICU nurse and the head of respiratory therapy in their green scrubs. They were two of many who cared for Elizabeth in her most critical hours. It was strange seeing each other outside the ICU setting, but when we recognized each other, we stopped to talk.

"Can you *believe* Elizabeth survived such a week?" I asked.

"No, it's amazing!" said the nurse. "We didn't think she'd make it through her first critical day. People as sick as Elizabeth normally don't survive."

"It was all that prayer that kept her alive," added the respiratory therapist. "Her survival through this week proves that God is the boss!"

As we spoke, we were unable to wipe the smiles of amazement off our faces.

"But why would we want to?" I asked myself.

We were united in delight! Their warm smiles and passionate remarks filled me again with fresh wonder.

"Lord, this feels incredibly good! Thank you *so much*!" I prayed silently after they left.

When Matt and I spent time with Elizabeth that morning, we noticed the swelling of her face and body had begun to subside. She looked more like her normal, beautiful self. We felt sure those who'd seen her earlier in the week would be happy to see the change. We certainly were.

The waiting room filled once again with McGovern supporters. Relatives from all over Southern California made the drive. Local friends and Biola friends joined family in loving reinforcement. Their presence brought us added strength.

However, I did notice a few people came with fear faces. Their ability to hope in such an impossible situation seemed small or non-existent. I realized I had to ignore their looks or comments. To remain strong and face the day, I had to focus only on words of faith we took in regularly from God's Word and through His mature, committed believers who made up the majority of our visitors. At any given time, we were walking either in faith or in fear. Both positions were mutually exclusive. If we gave in to fear, despair, or hopelessness, even a little, it was as if we fell into a jagged crevice far below us.

Elizabeth remained in the drug-induced coma, but the nurse informed us that any interested relatives could suit up and visit in her room. Those who didn't want to go in could remain in the hall outside and see her through the huge window looking into her room. So Elizabeth's grandparents and Aunt Jeri were able to spend a little time with their beloved granddaughter and niece.

Earlier a nurse had told us we could play CDs in Elizabeth's room, as long as they weren't too stimulating. So we brought in her favorite CDs, as well as a CD of soothing harp music. We omitted any that might be too loud or lively. Her nurse had already turned on the harp music as I went to visit her alone later that morning. I found it lovely and relaxing and it also took the edge off of my own unnoticed stress. After a while, one exceptionally beautiful song played. I'd heard it before, but I couldn't "name that tune." Later I discovered the name—Pachelbel's *Canon In D Major*.

As I listened to this majestic music, my thoughts turned to John and Elizabeth. They'd dated for a year, and you could tell they meant a lot to each other. As I stood beside Elizabeth's bed while the song played, all of a sudden I had a daydream. I saw John and Elizabeth and it was their wedding day. Pachelbel's *Canon in D Major* played as bridesmaids walked up the aisle. The wedding I saw was very God-honoring, and I sensed extraordinary joy. That glorious, lovely vision moved me deeply.

"What am I doing thinking about this right now?" I asked myself, snapping back into reality.

After all, this past Christmas John had given Elizabeth cute frog socks with squeaky toes as a gift. She loved them, but we didn't see marriage plans on the horizon.

One challenge the medical staff faced in Elizabeth's care was handling her tendency to become easily agitated. It didn't take much to elicit major reactions from her. Even opening and closing the sliding door of her room would do it.

I remembered an incident that took place four days earlier. A nurse noticed Elizabeth's head had started to slide off the pillow somewhat and the ventilator tube down her throat looked a little crooked. So she carefully picked up Elizabeth's head and moved it over on the pillow ever so slightly.

Then she barely adjusted the ventilator tube. Those small readjustments generated a huge response from sleeping Elizabeth—"Sleeping Beauty" as her Aunt Jeri called her. She reacted like she'd run laps or exercised vigorously.

For days Elizabeth had remained quite irritable when moved. Even so, the medical staff went forward with their weekend project of giving her a bath. While they bathed her, they encountered the problem again. Just having her body moved overstressed her taxed system. The numbers on her monitor spiraled downward from good to bad. They felt they lost a little ground just by doing general maintenance on her that day. And Elizabeth's anxiety level made it necessary to sedate her more than they wanted to.

For the past six days, everyone asked: "How did she get this?" Still, no one knew. Elizabeth didn't catch it from anyone at school, and no one close to her caught it from Elizabeth.

"How *did* she get this?" I wondered.

―――

By Sunday morning, Dr. Abergel sensed prayer had made a big difference in Elizabeth's survival. All along, as he'd listed off his desires for her improvement during updates, I'd turn them into specific prayer requests to give to our prayer supporters. That morning, in ICU, the doctor prefaced each item with the phrase "we can pray…" I was delighted to hear Elizabeth's doctor talking about prayer!

In our morning update, he also asked us to pray for the patient in room #157—two rooms down from Elizabeth's. He wanted us to pray she'd have a nice recovery and a good night's rest. He felt very tired. If that patient improved, he could get a night off.

A little later, I heard Dr. Abergel enthusiastically boasting to another doctor about the way our prayer support was helping our daughter. He said he'd tell Matt and me what Elizabeth needed for the day, and we'd pray for it. We got word out and many other people prayed for it, too. Then I heard Dr. Abergel tell him, "It's the best medicine!"

I prayed for Elizabeth outside her room that morning. Afterwards, I moved two doors down and prayed outside room #157.

Whenever Dr. Abergel reported any improvement, I tried to give God credit for His answer to our prayers for that exact request. But since ICU doctors may move on to another patient in a flash, I learned I had to be quick to mention God at work.

We were full of gratitude for everything the Lord had done that week. We felt hungry for worship and fellowship. After spending time in Elizabeth's room, we left and drove to church. As we entered the bright white sanctuary and sat alongside God's precious believers on burgundy-colored pews, I was surprised how right it felt to be there.

The leaders began to lead us in worship. One of the songs we sang was "Great Is Thy Faithfulness." While singing, I became aware those words perfectly showcased God's work in our lives over the past week. Morning by morning, we'd seen new mercies. The phrase "All I have needed Thy hand hath provided"[7] really touched me.

"Yes, Lord—that's exactly what you've done!" my heart cried, full of adoration. "All Elizabeth needed, your hand had provided. You're so awesome!"

Without any self-consciousness, I raised my hands up toward heaven as I sang, (which was totally uncommon for me).

Then the last verse of that hymn brought to mind other cherished gifts the Lord had faithfully given us during the week.

"Pardon for sin and a peace that endureth. Thine own dear presence to cheer and to guide. Strength for today and bright hope for tomorrow. Blessings all mine, with ten thousand beside!"

I felt as if my entire being wanted to acknowledge the truly great faithfulness of my God. The worship music profoundly affected me that day.

The entire service blessed us richly. When it was over, we returned to the hospital. It was almost lunch time, so I sent Maggie and Sarah off for Chinese take-out lunches while I stayed to visit with my youngest sister, Carol, who had just arrived.

So much had happened to tell Carol about. I started bragging about all God had done to help Elizabeth and heal her in the past week. One story after another came to me. I felt like a "motor-mouth"!

"Oh, have you heard about this?" I asked.

Then I told the story.

---

7   From the hymn, "Great Is Thy Faithfulness" by Thomas O. Chisholm. ©1923, Ren. 1951 by Hope Publishing Company, Carol Stream, IL 60188. All rights reserved. Used by permission.

"Here's something else unbelievable…" I said, starting the next story.

My words overflowed and I couldn't stop. My spirit rejoiced in God, my Savior. I had so much fun giving glory to God!

Maggie and Sarah returned with lunch, and Matt appeared in the waiting room just in time to share the meal with us. Then one by one, we opened our fortune cookies. When I cracked mine open, I noticed a wad of papers inside.

"Hey, what's going on inside this cookie?" I wondered.

My cookie contained five individual fortunes folded together instead of one. When we all saw the wad in my cookie, we found it incredibly funny and laughed like fools. It felt good to laugh so hard. It released a lot of tension.

In one way or another, we saw many ways my fortunes fit our circumstance.

- "Your efforts are budding—results will appear soon."
- "To reach distant places, you have to take the first step."
- "A cheerful letter or message is on its way to you."
- "Do something unusual tomorrow."
- "Everything will now come your way."

After Carol left, Matt and I went in for another visit with Elizabeth. We saw Dr. Abergel as we were leaving, so we talked with him briefly at the desk. He took a little time to share his passion for work with ARDS (Acute Respiratory Distress Syndrome). Then he told us Elizabeth had as complex a case of it as a person could get. We felt grateful, again, for his expertise.

Elizabeth still had occasional bouts of sepsis, so when problems developed, the medical staff responded quickly. Dr. Abergel anticipated new problems.

"She'll have ups and downs every day like a roller coaster," he said. "This is just maintenance."

Problems and challenges at that point didn't alarm him.

Seeing the doctor's calmness as he spoke about Elizabeth was wonderful. It meant he wasn't tremendously concerned for her survival.

Actually, "calm" was a word I'd usually use to describe Elizabeth. She was the calmest person in our family. One of her favorite, peaceful activities was reading. She loved it. I remember her reading one day when she was home between work and classes during her community college years. I wanted to ask her something, but I couldn't find her in the house. At the end of my search, I found her out on a porch bench at the front of our house, reading. The sweet fragrance of our gardenia bush in bloom near the bench wafted around her, enhancing her joy of reading and relaxing. She soaked up the sunshine and fresh air while her mind absorbed the contents of her book.

Maggie had been with us for a full week, but she had to get ready to take her final exams. With a heavy heart, she prepared to head back to school. John had a lot of school work ahead of him, as well, and had to drive back to Biola that night. And Sarah tried to adapt her thinking to return to a full day of high school the following day. Matt and I knew we'd miss them all terribly.

But Elizabeth's progress that weekend had lifted our spirits. An e-mail from Mary sent to Elizabeth around that time spoke to our hearts, too:

"The work the Lord is doing around and through your illness is amazing. Rejoice knowing that your illness and suffering has brought more glory to God than I could have imagined. Great is the Lord and most worthy of praise, His greatness no one can fathom. I love you, Elizabeth, and I can't wait to hug you and celebrate with you all that the Lord has accomplished in the last week. Peace be with you, dear sister."

CHAPTER EIGHT

"How Long, O Lord?"
(Psalm 13:1a)

For days, work had been ongoing to gradually wean Elizabeth totally off the paralysis medication that kept her in the drug-induced coma. When she woke up and noticed her surroundings, it was essential that she also remain calm. If she became anxious, they planned to sedate her with less intense medication. She finally reached the goal. Still, she continued to sleep all night and day.

After the update that morning, Matt left the ICU to make a phone call. I stood for a few moments outside Elizabeth's room and looked through the window at her and her monitor. Suddenly her eyes opened and looked greatly alarmed. She raised up both of her knees and her arms frantically flailed in the air. Her heart rate shot up from 92 to 144 within seconds.

I ran to the nurse's break room in a panic and alerted them to what had happened. Her nurse put down her cereal bowl and rushed into Elizabeth's room. I suited up quickly and went to her bedside.

The nurse wasn't too surprised Elizabeth woke up, but the medical staff didn't want her to move like that. She needed sedation, so the nurse left to get a shot.

I stayed by Elizabeth's bed. She looked at me with huge eyes that urgently spoke volumes.

"What's happening?! Why is all this stuff attached to me? Come on, Mom. Help me get out of here!"

I tried to calm her down.

"I'm here, Elizabeth," I said in a soothing voice. "You're okay. They'll help you."

She looked at me again with anxious eyes that urged me to take action on her behalf. Her face had a pained expression as she mouthed a word around her ventilator tube.

"Mom!"

Her silent, mournful moan grabbed my heart.

"I'm so sorry, Elizabeth," I thought. "I can't help you the way you want me to."

The nurse returned and gave Elizabeth a shot. A few moments later she'd fallen asleep again.

As a parent, I had a different perspective than the medical staff. For me, looking into Elizabeth's beautiful brown eyes again that day after seriously considering the possibility of her death was thrilling! It proved she was still with us. We could somehow relate to her. We could tell her again how much we loved her. We could share life together. I loved it!

In no time, her heart rate slowed down and, as a precaution, they loosely strapped her arms down to the sides of her bed.

I wondered when I would look into my daughter's eyes again.

Over the past four days, Elizabeth had made significant progress. I needed to tell some friends. I decided to call Joy, a good friend and Bible study leader, ten minutes before I knew the leaders' meeting would begin. After greeting my friend, I jumped right in with my first enthusiastic pronouncement.

"The doctor said Elizabeth now has a 90% chance of survival," I said.

"Oh, wow—can you hold on just a minute?" asked Joy, instantly excited by the news.

In the background, I heard her repeat my news to the other leaders.

"Yeah!" shouted the delighted prayer warriors.

Joy returned to the phone.

"And, Joy, she's progressed to the 45% level of oxygen support, which is 'Out of the danger zone,'" I said.

"That's so great!" said Joy, as the celebrative mood increased. "Just a minute, Diane."

Again Joy reported my news to the leaders. The uproar continued with more exuberant cheers in the background.

I paused and waited to hear Joy's voice return to the phone.

"And this morning, Elizabeth woke up briefly for the first time," I said.

Joy inhaled at the wonder of it all.

"Hold on, I'll tell the women," she said.

She told them what I'd said and, again, I heard more excited yells through the phone.

As my report ended, I realized phone rejoicing brought magnificent joy!

I was so thankful for all the precious women in that class. I wanted them to know their strong prayer support "availed much." I knew they'd keep at it.

Elizabeth awoke and reacted so suddenly that morning, I hadn't thought about what she was experiencing. A little later the nurse explained it to me.

"When patients like Elizabeth wake up, they encounter a whole new, confusing life," she said. "Their physical condition has been highly altered. It's shocking to them. They have no idea how long they've been in the hospital, what day it is, or if it's day or night."

When Matt returned to the ICU, I told him that Elizabeth woke up. The nurse began to teach us the best ways to communicate with her. First, she told us what not to say.

"Don't tell her anything upsetting," she said. "Don't tell her how long she's been in the hospital. Don't tell her she almost died."

It seemed Elizabeth only had ears for one conversation category—encouragement. Since anything we said could discourage her, frighten her, or decrease her sense of well-being, we had to mentally sift through all communications beforehand. It felt like we needed to play a game where the object was to exclude certain often-used words or phrases. Realizing our presence and attitudes could affect Elizabeth in such a strong way felt like both a privilege and a burden. We figured it would take real work.

Matt and I went back out to the waiting room to visit a friend who'd stopped by. I returned to visit Elizabeth alone before lunch and she opened her eyes again. She quickly became agitated and mouthed the word "Mom" a few more times, like she did earlier.

My heart ached.

"Calm down, Babe," I said. "You'll be okay."

But I was no help. She desperately wanted to be free of all the equipment hooked up to her body. She just couldn't lie there peacefully. The nurse gave her another shot and, in no time, she went back to sleep.

The nurse said they needed to finely tune the amount of sedatives they gave Elizabeth. They realized they were creating drug potency problems sedating her more often than they wanted to.

The doctor explained that young people use up the potency in sedatives and pain medicine quickly. Then they build up a tolerance to them. It's possible for them to use up a four-hour dose in only one to two hours. If older patients took the same amount of drugs Elizabeth had received, they'd sleep for days. Even with all she'd been given, she kept exhibiting anxiety. She became reactionary with the slightest provocation.

Another dependency problem develops when lungs in Elizabeth's condition receive large amounts of assistance from ventilators for a long time. It causes lung muscles to atrophy. Ventilated lungs get lazy and don't want to do their job. If they could speak, they'd probably say:

"I've got it made here with this ventilator doing all the work. This is so much easier than it used to be! I can relax all day. Ahhhh!"

Pulmonologists have developed various types of stress tests or physical therapy for lungs in this condition. During a stress test, Dr. Abergel would watch the patient carefully while forcing them to breathe on their own as much as possible. Early in the morning he liked to exercise their lungs for ½ hour at a time. Then he let them rest. Stressing the lungs this way made them stronger.

Now that Elizabeth was awake, he wanted to start stress tests with her to get her ready for extubation day, the day they would remove ventilator assistance for good. That would be her next big step, and Dr. Abergel believed she'd be ready for it soon.

Doctors look for signs from patients that prove their readiness to get off the ventilator. First, of course, their bodies require less oxygen assistance. Patients usually get off the ventilator at or near the 30% oxygen support level. Most reach that point within two weeks. Next, it's crucial that they be awake, alert, and able to function without sedatives. Third, the patient must have a cooperative attitude. Fourth, it's necessary for them to be able to cough and clear out their own lung secretions. And lastly, they must be able to forcefully inhale oxygen and exhale carbon dioxide.

Dr. Abergel said patients usually just got to a point one day when they were ready to breathe without ventilator assistance. The tube was taken out and the patient did fine. We all kept hoping that day was near for Elizabeth.

Elizabeth had been on a ventilator for about one and a half weeks. Usually a patient in her condition receives a tracheotomy after two weeks. It's a minor surgery in which a new opening is cut in the trachea and a smaller ventilator tube is inserted and sutured in place just after the larger ventilator tube is removed. A tracheotomy provides a more secure airway for the patient. It's less traumatic and makes the patient much more comfortable while remaining on the ventilator. With a tracheotomy, patients can take smaller steps toward extubation.

However, Dr. Abergel chose to hold off on giving Elizabeth a tracheotomy. He felt she was so close to extubation. He preferred giving her a chance to get off the machine completely when they thought she could sustain it. She currently sustained the 40% oxygen support level and they thought she'd probably move to the 35% level soon.

On her first day of wakefulness, Elizabeth also slept off and on since she required sedation regularly. By the time Matt and I went to dinner, she was asleep again. She woke up when we were gone and began looking around anxiously.

A nearby respiratory therapist sensed Elizabeth wanted something. She moved closer to talk to her.

"What do you want?" she asked simply.

Then she realized Elizabeth probably had no way to communicate. She wasn't sure if Elizabeth could move her hands or not, but she gave her a clipboard with the alphabet on it.

"Point to the letters in the word you want to spell," she said.

So Elizabeth lifted her hand and plopped it down. Her hand landed on the letter "n." She made many more attempts, probably aiming for other letters. But after every effort, her hand ended up on the letter "n." The clipboard and alphabet brought her only frustration.

Dr. Abergel was scheduled later that day to begin a two-week rotation at the Oxnard hospital. That filled both Matt and I with dread and fear of the unknown.

"He's such a good doctor," Matt said on the way to the hospital. "The thought of switching to another one makes me nervous for Elizabeth. What will happen when he's gone next week?"

Neither of us had a clue. We really felt we needed him to stay on her case. It didn't make sense to us for the doctors to switch in the middle of critical cases.

The thought of Dr. Abergel leaving sadly floated across our minds off and on throughout the day. Since we'd gone through so much together, we felt quite a strong bond with him.

Then the Lord nudged a question into my mind.

Are you trusting more in this doctor or in Me?

That was a big question. I knew I trusted God. He'd chosen to keep my daughter alive. But now He was asking me to examine my heart again.

"Am I trusting this doctor more than God?" I asked myself. "Well, am I?"

I continued to think about it, and I had to admit I was. I kept seeing a short drama play out in my mind.

It began with Dr. Abergel walking toward the ICU door to leave on his final night.

"I must stop him—we need him here!" I think as I run behind him.

I reach out and grab his arm, but he pulls away and keeps moving. He knows he has to leave and that his schedule is not determined by emotional outbursts from family members of patients. So I fall to the floor and begin to cry.

"Please don't leave us!" I plead.

But he keeps moving toward the door. I reach for his legs and manage to grab a hold of a foot, desperate to stop him.

"Please don't leave us!" I cry desperately. *"Don't leave us!"* I scream.

He drags me behind him for a few steps before he frees his foot from my death grip. Then he walks out the door.

I loved how honest my God was, even when I was wrong. He faithfully worked to set things right. He kept working in my heart that day. Because He's Almighty God, He won't accept anything from me but complete trust. He never meant for us to trust people more than Him. So I asked God to forgive what had developed in my heart. I remembered we began our time with Elizabeth in ICU, totally and utterly dependent on God to heal her.

When Matt and I talked about this struggle again later that night, we knew there was no other way but to continue on for as long as it took. We recommitted ourselves to fully trust God alone to provide all Elizabeth needed.

Not everyone close to Elizabeth saw her the day she first opened her eyes again. John was one who missed it. She'd been awake off and on for a couple of days when he came to visit. Tears filled his eyes at the joy of seeing her eyes opened again. We could tell they were both so happy to "see" each other again.

Through these critical days, God had been moving in John's heart and mind, showing him how much Elizabeth really meant to him. His feelings had grown deeper.

We left John in the room alone with Elizabeth that night. He was grateful for this because he wanted to reveal what was on his heart. During that alone time with her, tears once again filled his eyes.

"I love you," he said, to his Elizabeth.

He could tell she was coherent and that she knew what he'd told her.

Elizabeth began crying, too.

"I love you" were the next words she tried to form around the ventilator tube in her mouth.

John got the message. Even with all of the medical equipment between them, these two knew deep, romantic joy. John was so happy Elizabeth had shared what was also in her heart. God bound these two hearts together deeply, even in the midst of suffering.

"One day I'll be walking out of this hospital with all three of my daughters healthy," my dad heard me say when he visited earlier.

I'd pictured Elizabeth continuing to heal, getting off the ventilator, and leaving the hospital relatively soon. That was my plan. But by then, she'd been hospitalized for two and a half weeks and in the ICU for close to two of those weeks.

As we drove to the hospital that morning, we wondered if the doctor would tell us she was ready to get off the ventilator. Instead, the morning update revealed something else.

"Elizabeth's white blood cell count has gone up a little and her chest x-ray shows a worsening infection in her lungs," said the doctor. "She's developed a hospital-acquired infection called Pseudomonas. It's a bacterial lung infection—another pneumonia. This is a definite setback."

She'd been making good progress toward lower ventilator settings, but the work stopped because she was sick again. She needed rest. They planned to keep her at the current ventilator setting through the weekend, allowing her lungs time to heal.

However, the doctor gave us one encouraging tidbit.

"Bacterial infections are routinely fought by antibiotics," he said. "It's the viral infections that take over and do whatever they want for as long as they want."

Even so, it was very difficult for me to get it into my head that a recovering person in a totally isolated, germ-free ICU room could develop a new, additional illness.

I mean, the ICU had a high standard for cleanliness. The place was so clean, the floor was spotless and shiny bright. Each time we entered ICU, we were greeted by a fresh, antiseptic smell. We saw that undesirable items were disposed of quickly. As we visited in Elizabeth's room, we maneuvered around the cleaning staff often.

Questions began stabbing at my heart.

"If a person can't be protected there, where else can they go? How will Elizabeth ever get well if she keeps getting sick here?"

I was full of disappointment. I even wrestled in my mind with the phrase "hospital-acquired infection," because it didn't make sense to me. People go to the hospital to *un*-acquire infections, not to acquire more. I'd assumed a large measure of safety in ICU.

That morning I received an answer to prayer I wanted to reject.

You're going to have to wait.

God had the right to give me that answer, but I didn't like it at all. I was frustrated.

"I don't want to wait!" I thought.

God never promised a quick, easy exit from all difficulties, but my selfish nature wanted one immensely. I went out to a pretty patio area at the back of the hospital alone and sat and stared. I kicked seemingly unanswerable questions around in my mind. I mumbled a lot.

"What are we doing in this senseless place?" I asked out loud. "It's making Elizabeth sick!"

After a period of unproductive thinking, I was reminded again—thinking seriously about Elizabeth's situation was something I couldn't do for too long. I recalled a recommendation from J. I. Packer from his book *Knowing God* in his chapter about the adequacy of God.

> "Think of what you know of God through the gospel and apply it. Think against your feelings; argue yourself out of the gloom they have spread; unmask the unbelief they have nourished; take yourself in hand, talk to yourself, make yourself look up from your problems to the God of the gospel; let evangelical thinking correct emotional thinking.[8]"

God wanted me to move in that direction, so He provoked me to find Bible verses on "waiting" from my concordance. I got busy with that task. The verses I found were so good, I copied them down. Surprisingly, after I stepped out in faith, putting my mind where God wanted it again, I had a wonderful time in His Word. My God clearly and effectively communicates to the human heart. Here's one inspiring passage I found:

---

8   J.I. Packer, *op. cit.*, page 236.

> "I waited patiently for the Lord; He turned to me and heard my cry. He lifted me out of the slimy pit, out of the mud and mire; He set my feet on a rock and gave me a firm place to stand. He put a new song in my mouth, a hymn of praise to our God. Many will see and fear and put their trust in the Lord" (Psalm 40:1–3).

I was also encouraged to persist in trusting God by a quote I remembered from Brother Lawrence in his book *The Practice of the Presence of God*.

> "I do not pray that you may be delivered from your pains, but I pray God earnestly that He would give you strength and patience to bear them as long as He pleases."[9]

Refocusing again on God alone brought sanity and peace.

In less than a day, I'd begun struggling again with the difficulty of waiting for Elizabeth's recovery. For an impatient person like me, learning to wait patiently on God would require frequent and intensive training. As we left for home that night, we ran into Tami in the parking lot.

"Tami, Elizabeth has been hospitalized for two and a half weeks," I said. "I don't think I can take another two weeks of living like this! Her recovery is taking so long!"

Tami's response set me straight again.

"God is doing lots of work on all of us through Elizabeth's illness," she said. "He will take however long He needs to finish His work and fulfill His purposes for this situation. Many times, it's not just about someone being ill. God wants to change or repair other sick things in our lives. We need to trust that His work in His timing will produce very good things."

I became aware I had to let go of my personal time schedule for Elizabeth's healing and recovery. That was such a challenge! My focus during those weeks had been on Elizabeth and her problems. I had no

---

9 Brother Lawrence, <u>The Practice of the Presence of God</u> (New Seeds, Boston & London, 2005) #55.

idea of all the specific projects in each of our lives He planned to work on, but God did.

To achieve His current goals, the Lord allowed more suffering. It was open ended—we had no idea when it would be over. The life and death intensity of Elizabeth's first week in ICU had given way to a new form of suffering—facing slow progress, no progress, or setbacks. The change of pace from the first week was in stark contrast to the second week.

Even though it hurt, we sensed the presence of the Holy Spirit in us using the time to change and rearrange our hearts and priorities. In the process, our bond with each other grew deeper still.

Often we didn't notice changes in ourselves. Usually a family member would get a transformation glimpse, treasure it, and report it sometime later.

One day after lunch, when Maggie and I were walking back to the waiting room, she told me about new attitudes in her dad she'd seen developing.

"I've always loved the fact that Dad has been faithfully dedicated to 'be there' for his daughters," said Maggie. "It's easy to see that he loves Elizabeth, Sarah and me so much. But he's different somehow. Back on Day 1 when Elizabeth's life was so threatened, Dad seemed to realize everything was out of his control and it humbled him completely. That's when I began to see a whole new love, compassion, and tenderness in him. That first critical evening, he took the time to comfort Sarah and me and make sure we were both okay. While he comforted us, he gave us each a warm hug, but it was a new, more-loving type of hug."

Maggie took a few minutes to describe it to me. She said it began as just a normal hug, but then, without thinking about it, Matt's large, masculine fingers started to rapidly rub the middle of their backs up and down for a few minutes. He used a perfect balance between firmness and tenderness. They enjoyed it immensely. Since that time, Matt's "hug/backrub combo" has become a highly sought-after show of affection from him.

As we sat down in the waiting room, Maggie had one more thought about her dad to share.

"He's such a good dad," she added. "Now he more closely resembles a God-like father."

Maggie's report was so beautiful. Other family members had noticed it, too. So did I.

"Wow! This guy is so nice!" I thought, when I had spare moments to bask in the warmth of his changing heart. "I love seeing him this way!"

The next night, we decided to eat our fast food dinner at home for a change. Shortly after we ate, Elizabeth's absence made my heart ache deeply. Despair suddenly and mercilessly pounced on me and got a chokehold.

I went into my bedroom, kept the light off and fell onto my bed sobbing.

"Why isn't she better by now?" I wondered. "This is taking forever!"

The heaviness of the burden on my spirit was oppressive. It was so hard to continue in the situation with no end in sight. I felt sorry for myself.

"Lord, I can't bear this anymore!" I told Him again.

I cried and cried.

"What's going to happen?" I kept asking God. "How do we keep going like this?"

God didn't give me answers to my questions, but having a good cry was a huge relief. He soothed my broken heart and eventually gave me strength to get up off the bed and return to the hospital for an after dinner family visit with Elizabeth.

That night was the last night Elizabeth was under Dr. Abergel's care before he'd transfer for two weeks. Without knowing it, he gave his medical version answer to my urgent "how long?" question.

"I see Elizabeth being well enough to go home in two to four more weeks," he said. "Her chance of survival is 95%+ and her saturation numbers are at 93–95. Her lungs are starting to heal."

"How long will it be before she's ready to get off the ventilator?" Matt asked.

"Patients usually get to Elizabeth's point and are quickly able to get off the ventilator," said Dr. Abergel. "But she's not a usual patient. She moves at her own slow pace."

The doctor started to walk away. Then he turned and offered one final, hopeful comment.

"She's going to come out of this," he said. "For me, this is what's important—seeing patients like Elizabeth get better."

At the close of our talk, we realized it was time for him to go. God had been preparing us. We hated to see him leave, knowing he wouldn't be there the next day. But we thanked him profusely and said goodbye. Then we suited up for another visit with Elizabeth.

※

By that time, we'd become experts at donning the disposable gown, gloves, and masks every time we entered Elizabeth's room. We were adept at removing and depositing them in the trash can quickly as we left.

But as we thought about wearing our hospital garb, the mask was the item that caused us the most difficulty. It had to fit tightly over both the nose and mouth to protect us from Elizabeth's germs. There were two types of masks. The first was made of a soft substance like a thick Kleenex. It covered everything well and laid nicely over the nose and mouth.

The second type of mask had a rigid, pre-formed shape. The best thing about it was its pretty teal color. Both came in a variety of sizes. Sometimes the supply cart was fully stocked with all sizes and both types of masks. That assured us of a comfortable visit with Elizabeth.

At other times, the cart only had small sizes and our least favorite mask scenario—the stiff teal one. That particular mask actually felt like it was at least one size too small for all of us—one size does not fit all. Wearing any mask was very hot because we continually breathed in our own breath.

But the small teal masks caused us to calmly endure another form of discomfort. Once we'd wedged the small masks into position, they completely smashed our noses and pushed up our lips, scrunching them tightly together. The bottom edge of our noses touched our upper lips. Very little air could be breathed in. We had to work at breathing ourselves.

As we suited up that night, the small teal masks were the only ones available.

Matt was growing increasingly descriptive and funny through our hospital weeks. While we patiently began enduring them again that night, he started to see humor in those particular masks. He mentioned how uncomfortable he felt. He vividly described the nose and lip smashing feelings and how much the small mask restricted inhalation. There was only a thin slit between his lips through which air could be forcefully drawn in.

We each knew exactly what he was describing because we were doing precisely the same thing. We all burst out laughing. It was hilarious.

Talking cheerfully with Elizabeth when our mouths and noses were stuck in these positions was quite a task.

We were unaware that occasionally, Elizabeth's nurses also found the isolation gear challenging. Earlier that evening, before returning to Elizabeth's room, her nurse confided that his head was too big to wear the masks we were wearing.

"We hadn't noticed," I said.

So, just after our good laugh, Elizabeth's nurse entered her room wearing a huge get-up that made him look like a beekeeper. It covered his whole head and pumped a fresh air supply to him, which made us a little envious. However, with the air blowing around his face, he couldn't hear us very well. He looked at me.

"Am I talking too loudly?" he yelled.

"Yes," I said, nodding my head.

Mask humor in its many forms was quite amusing!

God had begun sending humor our way at random times and we noticed that it lifted our spirits. We found it to be a great coping mechanism. We welcomed it every time.

CHAPTER NINE

A Firm Foundation

When we entered the ICU the next morning, we discovered that the patient in room #157 had improved. We'd prayed for her, and she'd already come off her ventilator and was ready to leave ICU. I felt thankful she'd improved so much, but I also fought strong urges toward "getting-off-the-ventilator-quickly" envy.

We'd actually heard many varied comments about getting Elizabeth off the ventilator since she woke up from her coma. Each person on the medical staff had a strong opinion. Conflicting points of view were plentiful. So far, she'd been unable get off the ventilator in the usual way. But we were assured that there were many ways people got off ventilator support. For some, it's really easy. For others, it's quite a challenge.

That morning the infectious disease doctor determined Elizabeth was no longer contagious. She lifted the requirement for wearing gowns, masks, and gloves when we entered Elizabeth's room. *Free at last!* Now our noses and lips could return to their normal shapes. *Ahhhhhh!*

However, with the masks gone, our faces were completely exposed to Elizabeth. We needed to develop another skill quickly—presenting a neutral or encouraging face in her presence all the time, no matter what we felt inside. She remained very sensitive to our input in every way. If we were fearful, anxious, discouraged, or confused, we had to hide it from her. The unwritten motto we lived by in her room was: "Put on a happy face."

That evening, I visited Elizabeth alone while Matt and Sarah drove to Azusa Pacific to attend Maggie's final Concert Band performance for the semester. Elizabeth was sedated and resting. At about 6:00 I noticed her heart rate was 93, which was a good number. I'd learned by then that good numbers were our friends. I left for a dinner break, and while I was gone, Elizabeth's heart rate began going higher and eventually settled close to 120.

When I returned, I asked her nurse if I could go back into her room. She reported the higher heart rate and she seemed unsure. Then she remembered that many times the nurses had seen Elizabeth calm down, at least slightly, whenever family members were in her room, even if she was asleep. We saw it, too, especially at night. The nurse decided to let me return if I sat calmly. So I took a chair next to her bed and began to pray for her heart rate to slow down.

When I paused between prayers, I heard one of Elizabeth's Christian CDs playing softly on the other side of her room. I began to silently "sing in my spirit" along with it. It felt good to sing praises to God. I sensed the upward lift in my spirit yet again. Then I started praying again.

Suddenly an oversized "get well" card on the wall came loose and started to fall. On the way to the floor, it hit a large plastic "Wet Floor" hospital sign leaning against the wall directly underneath it. When the card hit the plastic sign, it fell and slapped the floor, making an extremely loud sound.

Just before the card fell, Elizabeth's heart rate had decreased from 120 to 113. After the noise, she didn't flinch and her heart rate didn't increase even one number.

"She's so calm!" I told God. "I'm amazed! Lord, I can't believe she didn't react to such a loud noise!"

God had cut her unusual sensitivity down. I stared at the 113 heart rate for many joyful moments and then I forged ahead in prayer for it to go even lower.

※

When people asked how they could help us, we usually drew a blank. So they searched for ways to support us. One wonderful couple brought us an awesome lasagna dinner one night. We were served with joy on the waiting room table. They made us feel like royalty. As God continued to stir people into action, we saw Him supply our needs lavishly!

Once the deacons at church saw Elizabeth's hospital stay lengthening, they told us they'd organize regular dinners for our family and have them delivered to our home. In no time, the first unbelievably good meal arrived. Then, day after day, magnificent meals graced our dining room table. We felt honored. We tasted the love and concern in every bite. We'd never eaten so well!

One friend included a large white envelope filled with a fresh batch of verses when she brought a meal. We devoured those like we did the excellent meal she provided. She knew feeding on God's Word again and again was required to stay strong. She reminded us to keep doing the right thing. God also urges us to demonstrate that devotion to His Word in scripture.

> "Let the word of Christ dwell in you richly as you teach and admonish one another with all wisdom, and as you sing psalms, hymns and spiritual songs with gratitude in your hearts to God" (Colossians 3:16).

Reading one verse occasionally would have led to spiritual starvation with the giant burden we carried. Since we tend to forget truth so easily, God didn't want us to let up on this activity.

In the Old Testament God instructed Joshua of the importance of this same spiritual discipline before he took on a new crucial role of leadership. Two verses in the book bearing his name encourage this.

> "Be strong and very courageous. Be careful to obey all the law My servant Moses gave you; do not turn from it to the right or to the left, that you may be successful wherever you go. Do not let this Book of the Law depart from your mouth; meditate on it day and night, so that you may be careful to do everything written in it. Then you will be prosperous and successful" (Joshua 1:7–8).

If God says to meditate on His book of the law day and night, how do we actually do that? Should we quit jobs, stop talking to family and friends and read our Bibles every waking hour? Of course not—but when it comes to boldly standing for God, we need routine spiritual nourishment. Whenever I skip time in God's Word, my faith grows weak.

Private time in the Word must be moved to one of the top priority positions on our "To Do" lists if it's not there already. In our busy lifestyles, it can be so easy to shorten or skip spiritual disciplines, but then we miss provision the Lord wants to give us. Scripture tells us there's no other way to get it.

> "It is written: 'Man does not live on bread alone, but on every word that comes from the mouth of God'" (Matthew 4:4 NASB).

Regular discipline in the Word helps to lay a foundation of faith and knowledge of God. It's best to lay that foundation before a crisis suddenly bursts on the scene. One wonderful pastor taught me that you have no more time to prepare for a crisis when it hits. It's too late to quickly get involved in an in-depth Bible study if you've neglected it for years. You go through the crisis on preparations made beforehand. The crisis either proves or disproves the soundness of your foundation up to that point.

From time to time on our journey, I considered the spiritual foundation the Lord had built in my life. I marveled at its sturdiness and beauty. It stood firm. Memories flooded in of those who'd labored faithfully to build that foundation as they served their God. Faces of dear Sunday school teachers I had as a child, camp counselors, pastors, leaders of my youth groups, Bible study teachers and leaders, and Biola College professors flashed across my mind. I also had fond recollections of favorite Christian musicians who'd encouraged my faith as I listened to their tapes and CDs at home and while driving in the car for years. The Lord had used all of them to lead me to Christ and help me grow in faith.

Later, as the Lord moved me into leadership in Bible study ministries, He'd used many edifying co-workers to keep me growing. Each of those people throughout my lifetime taught me to trust the Lord with my daily life and to know His ways. They taught me that walking in faith was life's greatest adventure. Matt and my daughters were blessed with similar believers who'd invested time and energy to build their faith foundations as they grew up. We were so grateful for them.

Some plant, others water. God causes the growth.

God continued to send His body to minister to us. Just one of many examples involved Sarah and her desire to attend her upcoming senior prom. One day when Jeri and I were talking, I mentioned Sarah's dilemma—no date, dress, money or time to buy a dress. Jeri felt led to be very available to our family during our journey.

"I've raised two sons and no daughters, said Jeri. "I never got to shop with girls. I'd be thrilled to go!"

Part of Sarah's journey through her sister's illness was having short bursts of extreme longing for life to be normal again. Since Matt and I were spending so much time at the hospital, Sarah found herself alone a lot. She felt uncomfortable in her unplanned independence. The days were very lonely for her. She felt so emotional at times, but she had no one at home to talk to. She lived with an intense, heart-pounding sadness.

When we talked about shopping for her prom dress, her first thought was that she wanted to shop with her sisters and maybe me. Then reality dawned on her.

"Oh yeah, things aren't the way I want them to be," thought Sarah.

After she adjusted to our new lifestyle again, Sarah began to look forward to her upcoming shopping trip with her Aunt Jeri.

Little did we know that Jeri and our sister, Nancy, had begun talking about the possibility of *buying* Sarah's prom dress for her as well. They'd mentioned the idea to a couple of mutual friends who began thinking about the plan, too.

The word "suction" became common during those days. Elizabeth no longer had the tight, silent breathing she had at the beginning. Now things were loosening up and she began coughing. Sometimes it was extremely painful. But with the ventilator tube down her throat, she wasn't able to get rid of mucus normally. They used a suction tube similar to the ones used by dentists. However, sometimes she needed help to remove mucus deeper in her lungs. So they had an extension attached inside the ventilator tube that went there and drew it out. The deeper suctioning looked quite unpleasant and it generated a lot more coughing. Sometimes she even appeared to be choking, but afterwards she'd feel some relief. Suctioning occurred many times a day, and it was difficult to watch.

One morning, after Elizabeth proved she understood conversations, a nurse asked her if she wanted her family in her room more often. She somehow indicated a "yes" answer, so we moved boldly toward that goal. Her concerned nurse also gave us a plea for more encouragement for Elizabeth. She told us the more Elizabeth was awake, the more she needed larger loads of encouragement. As Matt and I went in to visit, her eyes were open. We started encouraging her right away. We poured out cheerful, reassuring words.

"Elizabeth, you've been very sick, but you're getting better, I said. "In the hospital here, you're safe."

"The doctor and nurses are always carefully watching over you and working hard to help you get well," Matt added.

But our loving Lord knew that we needed encouragement for ourselves, too. That day as we left, we met a gift-bearing Tami in the parking lot. She handed me a set of small wooden stacking dolls from Russia.

"These stacking dolls can help you remember the principle that illustrates God's multifaceted work in our lives in all situations," Tami explained. "We can't see all the things God's working on, like the decreasingly smaller-sized wooden dolls hidden inside the original big one, but He sees it all."

Local friends realized we practically lived at the hospital by then, so they came there for updates. But as we began spending more hours in Elizabeth's room each day, people often couldn't find us. Some would leave disappointed without any new information.

There was a large, intense demand for daily updates. To meet it, I began writing one which included the latest specific prayer requests. I left it on a waiting room table, so people could get up-to-date details whether they saw us or not. Those written updates were a big hit. We noticed hospital staff members occasionally stopped and read them, too. People we didn't even know also rooted for Elizabeth to make it.

Since we spent so much more time together than normal, family members sometimes shared what God was teaching them in their quiet times. That was rich! And talking about what God was doing in our own lives was a pretty new occurrence for Matt and me as a couple. Growth was ongoing.

Friends told us we'd begun to boldly reflect God to others around us in a new way. Tami, for one, was quite observant. At one point she told us that watching the faith of our family increase caused the faith of others to increase also. She reported what she saw in an update to friends.

"Their faith is so evident. We see the Holy Spirit in them radiating out. They tell us God is their only lifeline. They are solid, steadfast on God. It's like this family is standing on a rock in the middle of a huge storm. The storm isn't over, but they are all okay because they are all huddling together on the rock. They are obedient to God's requirements to receive peace in their circumstances.

> 'You will keep in perfect peace him whose mind is steadfast, because he trusts in you' (Isaiah 26:3).

"I can see God's purpose in this being done. God is proving Himself to all of us. Besides working in Elizabeth's body, He's working to bring spiritual healing in many ways, which is always most important to Him. What God is doing with the McGovern family is incredible—beyond description. It's an honor to be a part of this."

We took no credit for those amazing, complimentary words. What people saw was God's strength and power alone. All glory belonged to Him for everything He did.

When a nurse told us that Elizabeth wanted her family to stay in her room more often, I knew it wouldn't be easy. During the first few weeks of hospital life, Matt and I really leaned on each other quite a bit. But he'd begun to feel he needed to return to work at least a couple of hours a day. Available hours from our support team were decreasing, not increasing. I had no idea how we could do what Elizabeth wanted. It overwhelmed me just to think about being Elizabeth's lone encourager for even part of the day.

"At the end of every day, I'm so tired," I told God. "Without help, I'm afraid I'll drown in this!"

Within a couple of days, Maggie's semester ended at APU and she returned home. She didn't have a summer job lined up yet, so she was available to help. She smoothly merged into Matt's partial vacancy on the support team. God faithfully provided a new, sufficient supply of help to meet the need, in the nick of time.

One evening before dinner, we had a surprise visit and update from Dr. Abergel. We were thrilled to see him since his schedule had him working in Oxnard, not in Camarillo. We were even more pleased to hear what he had to say.

"She's getting better. She's turned the corner and the lungs are healing," he said. "Even though it's a slow process, she *will* come out of this."

However, he did express confusion at why Elizabeth needed such an extremely high level of sedation.

"Is she a particularly anxious person?" he asked.

"No," I said. "She's normally very calm and level-headed. She's not given to hysterics or emotional outbursts."

—

Before we left for the night, one of Elizabeth's respiratory therapists shared a "getting off the ventilator" concern—her lung leaks. She said Elizabeth wouldn't ever be able to get off the ventilator unless the leaks were closed up.

We had no idea how lung leaks could be closed up. We'd heard staples or a very sticky glue type substance could possibly close them up. But those required the open lung operation, which Elizabeth couldn't tolerate. On the other hand, Dr. Abergel had said earlier that the leaks would never close up while she remained on the ventilator.

The respiratory therapist closed our conversation by telling us it was possible for the leaks to close up and heal on their own, but it wasn't likely. The lung leaks caused seemingly impossible prospects any way you looked at them. So we began to pray for God to handle another impossible task.

"If it's Your will, please close up the lung leaks."

—

In part because of the high sedation, we never knew how alert Elizabeth would be when we arrived. The next night when Matt and I went in for a nighttime visit, her eyes were wide open. We were so excited. It was the first time we both saw her so alert since she woke up. Eye contact with Elizabeth deeply moved us.

Out of the blue, my husband's inquiring mind wanted to see if Elizabeth knew what was going on. He told her to respond to his questions by blinking once for "yes" and twice for "no." Then he proceeded to ask her a string of questions.

"Do you recognize us?

Are your lungs hurting?

Do you know you're in the hospital?

Do you know you've got a breathing tube down your throat?

Do you know you're being well-taken care of by doctors and nurses?"

Elizabeth blinked her "yes" and "no" answers quite intelligently. The three of us were so happy to be communicating on some level. Matt and I were thrilled to see her respond. With each blink, we had more joy. Elizabeth was coming back to us. Her mind and memory seemed intact.

Matt's scientific nature constantly asks questions and seeks to discover facts. But I felt he was getting carried away with his question/blinking project.

"We don't want to wear out her blinking ability," I said. "Maybe you should stop asking her so many questions."

"I'm communicating with Elizabeth here," he replied earnestly. "I don't want to stop."

He asked Elizabeth one more question.

"Do you know we really love you very much?"

She blinked her eyes over and over again in response. It was a blink fest from Elizabeth. Matt and I found ourselves blinking back tears that came to our own eyes. We were ecstatic!

In the early weeks of her illness, Elizabeth had taken overdoses of drugs out of necessity. One ongoing project was to get her off of sedatives. The medications were strong, so they brought in a neurologist to oversee a slow, careful withdrawal just like drug addicts go through.

When she tolerated lower amounts of sedatives, it left her very sleep-deprived. All the sleeping she'd done earlier had been induced by drugs.

Now the question kept coming up: "What do you do with someone who can't sleep?"

On two different occasions, her night nurses answered the late night insomnia problem with hair styling. They each washed Elizabeth's hair and put it in braids. One male nurse made the first attempt, producing a lopsided set of braids. But a few nights later another nurse, one who knew how to put in beautiful French braids, did a nice job. Elizabeth looked quite lovely when we saw her the following morning.

Before Dr. Abergel rotated to the hospital in Oxnard, he informed us that Elizabeth would need physical therapy.

"When the human body, young or old, remains totally inactive for even one and a half weeks, muscles really atrophy," he said.

Just recently Elizabeth's physical therapy had begun on her legs, feet, toes, arms, wrists, and fingers. Sessions weren't long, but they were challenging. We were thankful her muscles responded well and improvements showed up relatively quickly.

About that time, Elizabeth's eyebrows became a very strong communicative tool. Sarah discovered one particular gesture and named it "Hi eyebrows." When Elizabeth made "hi eyebrows," she raised both eyebrows and opened her eyes wide. She greeted loved ones that way as they entered her room. We all interpreted her gesture to mean: "Hi, I'm happy to see you!" Communication from Elizabeth returned in slow, subtle ways and every tiny form was precious to us. She blinked her eyes and mouthed words. After her arms got a little stronger, she pointed. We all longed for improved conversations. We missed her so much and we wanted her back in every way. Early on, when we attempted to understand Elizabeth's gestures or mouthing of words, it felt like we were playing a game of charades. She was so happy when one of us got it right. She enthusiastically raised those eyebrows and nodded for "yes."

By that time, Elizabeth had been in the hospital a little over three weeks. She'd been in the ICU eighteen days. When we saw that particular late afternoon turn calm and restful for Elizabeth, Matt and I decided to go ahead and go out on a date. It was the day of our 25th wedding anniversary. We wanted to go out for dinner that night.

Before the health crisis, we'd planned to spend the weekend at a beautiful bed and breakfast near Monterey, California to celebrate our significant life event. After Elizabeth got so sick, Matt cancelled our reservation, figuring we'd celebrate later.

We went home that evening to get ready to go out. As days had turned into weeks, we'd begun to feel worn out. It was a new kind of intense exhaustion. Each day by bedtime, our physical energy levels plummeted totally. Because of our wearied bodies, we felt somewhat like we were simply going through the motions that evening.

But I'd been learning to rejoice in the simple things. I was happy just to ride with Matt in the car. I even found it strangely exhilarating to sit close to him in a restaurant instead of a hospital.

We'd agreed beforehand that we wouldn't talk about Elizabeth while we were out. Conversation started with mindless chatter. We found, again, that it was extremely difficult to switch gears. We found it easier to turn off words than to turn off thoughts.

Eventually, we succeeded at talking about a non-Elizabeth topic.

"I wish things were different and that we were eating dinner at a restaurant in Monterey instead of here," Matt said. "Remember our first anniversary in Monterey when I golfed on the Pebble Beach golf course and you drove the golf cart?"

"Oh, yeah—that was fun!" I said. "What a beautiful place! Each time I drove the cart to a new hole, it was like God displayed a new piece of His magnificent artistry before my eyes. Lush green, manicured lawns within lavish landscapes led to exquisite views of the Pacific Ocean and its shoreline. Occasionally I saw otters in the bay floating comfortably on their backs digging crabs out of their shells. All of the scenery was really something."

Even though we'd both grown up in Southern California spending lots of time at the beach, as young adults, we were still irresistibly drawn to its breathtaking beauty. It never gets old! Being near the ocean in Monterey was the perfect place to celebrate our anniversary.

We'd been blessed to take many nice weekend trips through the years as a couple. Before our food came that night, we went on talking about other favorite spots like Yosemite and Laguna Beach where we'd shared special memories. Sometimes the best we could do when the kids were small was to go out for a nice dinner as a couple. We were grateful for each anniversary getaway.

To commemorate our 25th year, we enjoyed an excellent barbeque rib dinner at a local restaurant. Then, we read anniversary cards with mushy notes inside, and gave each other gifts before we returned to the hospital. As the evening drew to a close, I was full of gratitude.

"Lord, I'm so thankful for Matt's faithful commitment to me. When we really work together and love each other properly, we're such a great combination of personalities and abilities. You knew what You were doing when you brought us together. You've carried us through 25 years since May 5, 1979—the happy ones, sad ones, and all those in between."

We'd named our greatest joys from our marriage Elizabeth, Maggie, and Sarah.

CHAPTER TEN

"I Love Jesus—He Is My Strength"

THE NEXT DAY THERE WERE no new traumas or procedures for Elizabeth, so Maggie and Sarah came up with an idea. Earlier, we'd all noticed how much it refreshed Elizabeth to have her hair washed. Female patients found it particularly invigorating. Another neglected grooming project was shaving her legs. Hairy, unshaved legs were particularly bad because they were often exposed. Elizabeth's were in desperate need of a razor.

Maggie and Sarah checked with the nurses about their plan. Then, they ran it by Elizabeth, and she gave her raised eyebrow, nodding approval. They gathered a razor, shaving cream, and a big bowl for water from home and set out to shave their sister's legs.

Because Elizabeth's limbs were still very weak and heavy, Maggie and Sarah took turns lifting and gently manipulating each leg as the other shaved the overgrown hair. It took quite a while, but they did a great job. It was a nice gift to Elizabeth.

The shaving sisters were proud! Nurses and respiratory therapists who went into her room afterwards admired them as much as we did. Some even gave her legs that quick "wow, they're so smooth!" rub. Maggie is our family hairstylist, manicurist, and fashion consultant. After Elizabeth's legs were done, she planned to manicure all of Elizabeth's nails as well.

With Elizabeth all primped and polished, the four of us relaxed in her room and listened to The David Crowder Band. Just then, a song with a fun beat and the catchy phrase, "Nah nah nah nah nah nah—Hey!" began to play. We saw Elizabeth moving her recovering feet and hand muscles to the beat of the song. She raised her feet and dropped them quickly with the beat when the word "hey!" came in. Her fingers responded to the beat, too.

"You go, girl!" said Maggie, as she watched Elizabeth.

We all laughed. It felt good to smile at each other and dance around to the music.

During those hospital weeks, Matt discovered his own way to meet a specific need for Elizabeth. Fevers warmed her up and, at times, the room was hotter than usual. When he first arrived in her room, he'd greet her and then ask if she wanted a cool washcloth on her forehead. If she did, he'd soak one in cold water from the sink in her room and lay it on her forehead.

Maggie, too, provided a unique service for Elizabeth. Because her mouth remained slightly open all the time, small amounts of drool turned hard and crusty at the corners of her mouth. It grew annoying for her. Maggie wiped away the crusty drool and any sticky goo that was there. Sometimes she also applied soothing lip balm on the dry areas afterwards.

It may have been a disgusting task, but she could tell Elizabeth placed high value on the assistance. Whenever Maggie entered the room, Elizabeth looked at her with great enthusiasm because she knew "corner of the mouth" help had arrived.

And Matt discovered an additional form of Elizabeth assistance. One day, he saw that one of the chest tubes was clamped down by a bar at the side of Elizabeth's bed. It restricted necessary suction, which could cause her lungs to collapse again. He quickly reported it to the nurse. After his discovery, Matt took it upon himself to inspect her chest tube equipment every time he entered her room. He also made sure things appeared to be draining right. If he noticed anything unusual, he pointed and asked questions. It was a good thing Matt was on the job.

The next morning was Mother's Day. Maggie and Sarah got up early and brought me breakfast in bed. Sarah shaped scrambled eggs into a heart on my plate that were accompanied by blueberry muffins and Earl Grey tea. Maggie made a pretty floral arrangement for me from blossoming bushes at the front of our house. The vase contained sweet-smelling roses, colorful bougainvillea leaves, and dainty night-blooming jasmines with their bold fragrance.

Both girls gave me sweet cards and some lovely perfume. They reminded me how much having them as my daughters blessed my life.

Later that morning, as Matt and I drove to the hospital, he was very quiet. I'd begun talking about the current concerns we had for Elizabeth—our new lifestyle. She was the topic of conversation 90% of the time. Matt rarely showed his emotions, but as we drove, his face grew sad and fearful. Suddenly, he burst into tears.

"What if she never gets better?" he asked desperately. "What will they do with her? What kind of life will she have?"

He pulled the car over to the curb. I moved closer and put my arm around his shoulder. Questions like those raced at us and tried to choke us at unpredictable times. I recalled being grabbed by similar questions a few days earlier. I had no new answers for him. I looked into the broken heart of a father who deeply loved his daughter. He felt helpless to fix the situation. He couldn't protect her from any of it.

I felt very close to Matt in those pain-filled moments. So much of the time during those days we were too busy to voice the deep fears in our hearts. And we knew we couldn't stay in the fear zone too long, anyway. He was so beautiful and tender in his agony. It knit our hearts together in a profound, new way as parents.

It's a sad reality that an inaccurate expectation has been put on men by our society. They've been told to shut off their deepest feelings for a lifetime. They're encouraged to "Show no weakness!" But in some situations, the only appropriate response is to cry and feel deeply. Strong and loving men are the ones who have done that. God's heart shines through them.

I gave Matt the same hopeful answers we'd given each other before. They were the same answers many other believers, who were full of faith, had shared with us from the beginning. "God can do impossible things. We will keep trusting Him. We will ask Him for more hope."

We had to keep looking to Him and not at the storm in our lives that still had not let up.

After Matt calmed down, he drove the rest of the way to the hospital.

For days, the abundance of "get Elizabeth off the ventilator" talk constantly surrounded her and anyone near her. That morning, we tried to encourage her to get ready emotionally and spiritually for that task.

During Elizabeth's illness, Matt was becoming more and more involved in the spiritual life of his family. He was beginning to take his leadership role more seriously.

On that Mother's Day morning, as I stood at the side of Elizabeth's bed, Matt comfortably took the lead and shared from one of his recent quiet times with her. As she grew up, she never mentioned him taking the initiative to do that before. That morning, she seemed to love it. He read an Old Testament story to her about Joshua and Caleb from Numbers chapter 13. They were two of the twelve Hebrew spies who bravely wanted to follow God's leading to go in and take the Promised Land.

> "Then Caleb silenced the people before Moses and said, 'We should go up and take possession of the land, for we can certainly do it'" (Numbers 13:30).

But many others put extreme pressure on them to ignore God's leading, focus on obstacles instead of God's abilities, and give up. Because the majority of people in the story distrusted God, they didn't achieve their goal. They wandered forty years because of it. Matt told Elizabeth she didn't want to do that with ventilator work. She needed to be brave and courageous.

Suddenly I realized something big had just happened. Many times before, I felt like I'd carried the major portion of the burden for spiritually training and encouraging our daughters. But when I saw him take the lead that morning, I experienced how good it felt to naturally share that burden. Pressure was gone and an awesome joy filled my spirit!

When Matt and I thought about Elizabeth facing the huge challenge of ventilator extubation, we remembered that she was a person who pursued the right direction wholeheartedly, once she knew what it was. Back in high school, we'd seen her persevering heart when she participated on the track team. She worked hard to build up stamina and learn new skills. And we always loved watching her run races as well as performing the triple jump. There was a beauty to it.

She even loved running as a young girl. I recalled the tradition our daughters started when they were little girls. At the end of a visit with their grandparents, they said their goodbyes at the house. Then they'd jog to the corner of the block of our street. They'd wait until their grandparents' car approached. Just when the car was in front of them, they'd wave enthusiastically and yell "goodbye" again. To Elizabeth, Maggie, and Sarah, this was the complete way to say goodbye and it was the most fun. Once the car was out of sight, the three of them raced back to our house as fast as they could. Elizabeth got there first every time.

She needed that same perseverance and drive now.

❦

Before Elizabeth became sick, she'd been waiting to hear whether or not she was accepted by graduate schools. She was interested in becoming a marriage and family counselor. Her top choice was a two-year program at Azusa Pacific University. If accepted there, she and Maggie planned to share an apartment together. Her second choice was a four-year PhD program at Rosemead School of Psychology, located at Biola University. Eventually, letters from the schools came in the mail.

We waited for the right time to have Elizabeth open them herself, but that time kept escaping us. Finally, we opened them for her and discovered she'd been accepted at both schools. We had some good news for her, but we wondered when we should tell her. We doubted she'd be out of the hospital in time to graduate from Biola that spring, much less start graduate school in the fall.

❦

A week earlier, Elizabeth had quickly recovered from the Pseudomonas and another doctor rotated in after Dr. Abergel left. The team of doctors consulted regularly on her case, and each of them had a unique perspective and specific concerns. The new doctor had a cautious approach. He felt the risk with Elizabeth was still high. He knew lungs took a long time to heal and he had wisdom to go slowly.

As he began his watch, his first concern was the continuing leaks at the top of her lungs. Chest tubes dealt with the excess air but didn't correct the root of the problem. Leaking air from her lung air sacs provided a constant source of other complications.

He also noticed her carbon dioxide levels were too low, and when he saw a tiny rim of air at the top of her left lung in an x-ray, he wondered what could be done about it. Elizabeth also relied heavily on pressure control from the ventilator, but her lungs needed to generate pressure on their own again. The doctor believed the lung leaks could close up over time if she'd require less pressure assistance. He knew when a patient got off a ventilator, the balance of many components had to be right.

Going at a slower pace with regard to the ventilator was difficult for all of us to accept. It felt like progress stopped. But when the doctor tried to make aggressive ventilator changes, her body wouldn't tolerate them. Again her numbers spoke for her body.

"If you go too fast, I could develop big problems. Go slowly with me."

So he cautiously worked to make subtle reductions. At times Elizabeth resisted even small changes. The medical team lived out the maxim: "If at first you don't succeed, try, try again."

Every once in a while, however, little improvements were made. After a week, the doctor realized that persisting with slow, small steps had begun to bring desired changes. As he prepared to rotate out, he mentioned specific, slight improvements and progress on his areas of concern. After talking again, he and Dr. Abergel believed a day would soon come when she'd be ready to get off the ventilator.

The challenge of getting Elizabeth off the ventilator was passed to the next doctor as he rotated in the next day. He was the senior partner in the group of ICU pulmonologists and had twenty-one years of experience. On his watch, he was the first to point out stiffness in Elizabeth's lungs—they didn't demonstrate the normal give and take of healthy functioning lungs. Pressure control also remained a big challenge for her to give up. Even so, he felt she wouldn't need a tracheotomy because she kept getting closer and closer to extubation day.

One day, he implemented another round of stress tests. He wanted to see how she'd do during brief periods off the ventilator. He said he'd be happy if she went five minutes.

On attempt number one, she went fifteen minutes! The attempt went well, but afterwards Elizabeth noticed a sharp pain in her left lung. She was told that her body would feel sensations she hadn't been feeling for a while. Exercising those inactive lungs caused pain. The doctor didn't seem worried about it.

Her second attempt off the ventilator lasted twenty-seven minutes. A little while later, they noticed Elizabeth's heart rate had gone higher. An hour or so after her second "workout," Elizabeth suddenly began choking. Her eyes bugged out and she began waving her hands and arms as if she couldn't get any air. Her heart rate went very high—up to 160. She looked scared. Her nurse called in a respiratory therapist who was able to help Elizabeth breathe. The issue was fully resolved after about twenty minutes. A chunk of mucus or something had clogged her tube.

Before leaving that afternoon, the doctor encouraged Elizabeth.

"Some things will hurt a little more when you work your lungs, but when you're done, it won't hurt anymore," he said. "You've got a great body that will tell you what it needs."

Later that evening, attempt number three was made. It lasted thirty-four minutes. Elizabeth seemed pleased to have increased her time with each attempt. It was awesome seeing her breathe the same air we were breathing. Her daily total off-the-ventilator time was one hour and sixteen minutes. But when they put her back on the ventilator, she looked very tired.

"What could that mean?" I wondered.

When we first entered ICU the next morning, Elizabeth's nurse looked tired and annoyed—and the day had only begun. She told us things just seemed to be bothering Elizabeth.

Earlier, she'd summoned someone in repeatedly and they hadn't been able to figure out how to help her.

They gave her the clipboard with letters again, encouraging her to try spelling out her words. Once again, it brought frustration. So the nurse set the clipboard aside. Then she checked to make sure her patient was as comfortable as possible and left her alone. Elizabeth was just having a crabby morning.

That morning Maggie wore a new Azusa Pacific University sweatshirt to the hospital. Elizabeth was determined to keep trying to get information. While I was absent from Elizabeth's room for a while, she began trying to get information from Maggie.

She started out by pointing to Maggie's new APU sweatshirt.

"Mom and Dad gave it to me for my birthday," Maggie said. "Isn't it pretty?"

Elizabeth agreed it was, but she seemed to want to know something else. A little later she pointed to the sweatshirt and then to herself.

Maggie began thinking hard, trying to figure out what her sister wanted to know.

"Oh, do you want to know how school is going?" Maggie asked.

No, that wasn't it either. Once more, Elizabeth pointed urgently to the sweatshirt and then to herself.

Maggie was developing strong intuition with Elizabeth in the ICU, but she was still racking her brain trying to figure out the mystery. It finally hit her.

"Do you want to know if you were accepted at APU?" she asked Elizabeth.

Elizabeth nodded "yes" with accompanying raised eyebrows and wide eyes.

"I'm not sure," said Maggie.

Maggie remained vague, telling Elizabeth she recently received letters from both APU and Rosemead School of Psychology. She carefully eased off the topic.

Later, when I heard of Elizabeth's eagerness for information about her life, I decided it wouldn't upset her by telling her good news. So we told her we'd read the letters. She was glad to hear that she'd been accepted by both graduate schools. The next time we went home, we retrieved the letters and took them to Elizabeth so she could read them herself.

That night we returned for the final visit with Elizabeth from 8:00 to 10:00 p.m. As we prepared to leave, Matt and I looked at her numbers and they didn't seem right to us.

"Matt, does something seem to be bothering her?" I asked.

"I was thinking the same thing," Matt said. "But what could be wrong?"

We had no idea, so we told Elizabeth goodbye for the night and stopped at the nurse's station on our way out.

"Can we call and check on Elizabeth a little later?" we asked the nurse.

"You can call any time you're worried," he replied.

We walked out of the hospital accompanied by a strange feeling and drove home. We kept discussing it as we got ready for bed. The unsettled feeling persisted.

At 11:30 p.m. Matt called ICU.

"Elizabeth pulled her ventilator tube out shortly after you left," said her nurse. "She's quite upset and crying a lot. You can come in and help calm her down, if you want."

Matt left immediately. As he drove back to the hospital, it made him sad to think about having to scold his daughter while she was so sick.

"How can I be gentle and 'get on her' at the same time?" Matt asked himself.

Whenever a patient pulls out a tube like that, the ICU staff waits to see how they respond, just in case they're able to sustain healthy breathing. Elizabeth lasted for a brief while, but the color in her face grew pale and they knew she needed to be re-intubated. The ER doctor was called in to do the job.

When Matt arrived, he put on calming music, sat close to Elizabeth, and held her hand for about an hour. He gently comforted his hurting daughter. Before he left, he briefly "got on her" about the tube.

"You shouldn't pull this tube anymore," he said calmly.

"I know," mouthed Elizabeth's lips around the ventilator tube.

Having that tube put back down her throat was painful and sad for her.

No one was sure whether she'd pulled the tube out accidentally or intentionally. After the incident, they strapped Elizabeth's hands tightly to the sides of her bed. The straps could be loosened if a nurse or family member was in her room with her.

When we entered her room the following morning, the nurse untied her hands. We knew Elizabeth was depressed by the look on her face. We all shared her disappointment.

Occasionally that day, Elizabeth moved one of her hands up to a position where she could easily grab the tube. I felt edgy. I was nervous she'd do it again. One time, I said something.

"Elizabeth, you shouldn't pull the tube," I said.

Then I moved her hand away from the tube and back down to the side of the bed.

"Mom, you're over-reacting!" said Maggie.

"Yeah," said Sarah. "You don't have to watch her hands like a hawk!"

Elizabeth, too, gave me some questioning looks. She didn't seem to understand why seeing her hand near the ventilator tube mattered so much to me.

"She won't do it again," Maggie assured me.

"How am I supposed to know that?" I asked myself.

Whenever Elizabeth was left alone in her room again, her arms were tied tightly. The medical staff felt it was necessary. She didn't seem to like it at all.

I hadn't participated in my morning Bible study for weeks, and the day came for the final leaders' meeting for the year. I'd always loved that ministry. I was so thoroughly taught God's Word and encouraged to grow in faith through the years. Serving in leadership with them was such a privilege. I'd missed them so much.

Maggie volunteered to take the majority of the day with Elizabeth all by herself so I could go. That freed me to get away without feeling I was abandoning Elizabeth. I hadn't been away from Elizabeth for that long in close to a month. I felt like I'd been in a cave for weeks. *Friends.* Surprisingly, socializing felt awkward.

Since Elizabeth's illness began, each of her family members always drew lots of attention when they were out. Friends quickly swarmed around us like we were celebrities, eagerly clamoring for an update on her condition.

"How's Elizabeth?" was the question we'd hear from all directions.

It was so good to know they cared and were praying, but it grew overwhelming.

"We're celebrities because we have a loved one in ICU—strange!" we thought.

However, we always had many stories and answers to prayer to talk about.

At the leaders' meeting, I wanted to blend in with the others. I hoped I wouldn't draw too much attention away from God's agenda for that day. God had done many beautiful things in the lives of the leaders and class members all year long and we wanted to share them all. But after four hours of fun and refreshing fellowship, I knew I needed to get back.

Back at the hospital, Elizabeth's improving condition was leading to some surprising new frustrations. We'd learned critical patients don't always wear undergarments, since every part of their anatomy had to be quickly accessible anytime. When performing therapy, the physical therapist brings small white towels to cover the patient's private areas, preventing them from worrying about unnecessary, embarrassing exposure.

Maggie and I were in Elizabeth's room during her physical therapy that afternoon. We saw the physical therapist cover Elizabeth well, but when he finished exercising one leg and started on the other, she became increasingly agitated. Elizabeth tried to point to what she needed, but the physical therapist couldn't tell what was troubling her.

Maggie had become very good at anticipating Elizabeth's needs. She spotted the edge of a towel under the leg Elizabeth had just exercised. The rest of the towel was in a wad under her leg making her uncomfortable. It was quickly removed and everything was o.k. again.

Later, a nurse had mistakenly left Elizabeth's hospital gown bunched under a leg after caring for her. She grew uncomfortable about that, too. Again, Maggie was wonderful with Elizabeth. She spotted the trouble and returned the nightgown to its "just so" position. By pointing and passionate gesturing, Elizabeth finally got people to understand how much those little things irritated her. That bright, active young woman grew increasingly frustrated having to remain mostly immobile and limited in her communication abilities.

As she cared for her sister, it was easy to see Maggie and Elizabeth had a strong, loving connection. Maggie "got" Elizabeth.

Spending a lot of time in Elizabeth's room also allowed Maggie to observe some of her sister's peculiarities as an ICU patient. One time she saw Elizabeth become upset because a nurse moved her bed diagonally for some reason. By gesturing, Elizabeth insisted her bed had to be exactly parallel to the walls of her room. Readjustments were made after the nurse left.

Another time Elizabeth worked hard to communicate her desire to have her bed in a sitting position. Adjustments were made to her bed, but she was fickle. Within five minutes in the sitting position, she wanted it back in the original position.

Sometimes, trying to help Elizabeth could hurt your feelings a little. If a series of communication attempts failed, she'd roll her eyes. That sent a message out of frustration.

"Never mind, you dummies."

"Ouch!" we thought.

However, family members saw Elizabeth working hard to come back to us. She created new gestures that got her messages across better. We learned that if she wiggled her fingers a certain way, it meant she needed someone to scratch an itch for her. If she pointed directly to her dad, it was her abbreviated request for wanting a cold washrag on her forehead. And if she demonstrated how well she could move her feet and squeeze her hands, it meant she was pleased with her physical therapy progress.

Elizabeth discovered a TV remote at the side of her bed. She was getting good at handling it. As her hands became stronger, her thumb grew powerful enough to push the "on" and "off" buttons. She liked the sense of control handling the remote gave her.

The next morning was the fifteenth day since she woke up from her coma. Her nurse sensed Elizabeth was still very eager to communicate. Once again, she handed Elizabeth the clipboard with the alphabet. Her nurse also gave her blank sheets of paper and marker pens in case she wanted to try writing letters on her own. Her hands seemed too weak to do that, but she tried a little. By the time Maggie and I arrived in her room a while later, Elizabeth was aggravated with the whole idea again. The items that were meant to help were set aside once more.

But as it drew closer to noon, Elizabeth pointed to the clipboard, paper, and markers again. I gave them to her.

I wasn't expecting much. I hoped she wouldn't get too upset if her efforts were thwarted again. I sat at the side of her bed and my eyes caught what she was writing. I stared at it, trying to determine what it said. It roughly looked like she'd written "Hi."

"Did you just write 'Hi'?" I asked her.

Elizabeth nodded.

Tears welled up in my eyes.

"Maggie, come see what Elizabeth wrote!" I said quickly.

Maggie got to the side of Elizabeth's bed in a flash. She loved seeing the word Elizabeth had written, too. She also began to cry.

Even Elizabeth had tears in her eyes. "Hi" had been difficult for her to get on paper, but she wasn't done yet. She kept writing. Maggie and I had our eyes glued to the paper.

"I love you," was Elizabeth's next message.

Maggie and I were thrilled. The words, tears, and amazement continued. Her capital letter "I" looked sort of like a Christmas tree, but her letters improved as she wrote more.

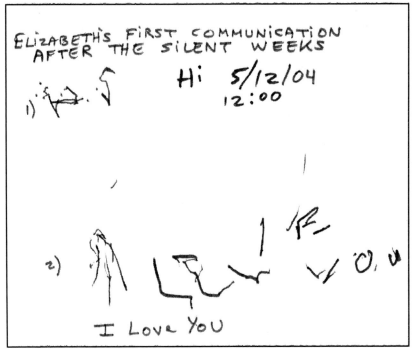

Elizabeth's first writing, part 1

Elizabeth completed her third message.

"I love Jesus."

Maggie and I were spellbound. Our hearts felt so powerfully and tenderly intertwined with Elizabeth's as we saw her communicate such precious words. Then she wrote another note.

"He is my strength."

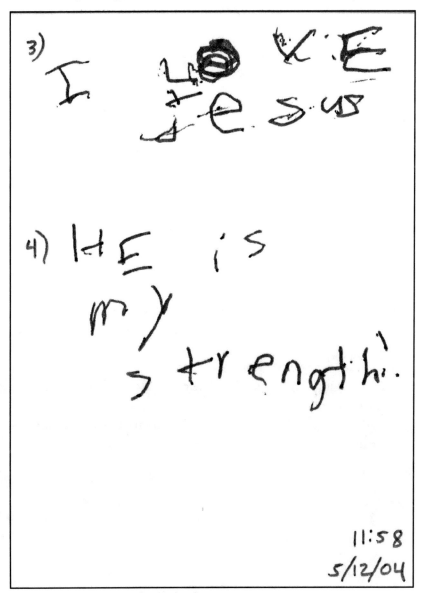

Elizabeth's first writing, part 2

Finally—a big breakthrough!!! We were so excited!!! Maggie and I felt blessed to be in Elizabeth's room at that time. We each hugged her carefully. We praised God for such a sweet surprise. Elizabeth was so happy to be able to share what was on her heart again!

This was the beginning of many more notes from Elizabeth. From then on, she could tell everyone exactly what she needed or thought. It made everything so much easier and quicker. Elizabeth was very relieved.

We couldn't wait to tell everyone else that she'd been able to write that morning. We especially wanted to share the beautiful words she'd just written.

Elizabeth's intense desire to communicate with us reminded me of the Heavenly Father's profound desire to communicate with people. He's always desired a deep sharing, a thorough knowing, our careful listening, and a close relationship unlike any other with His children. He persists in His efforts to develop vibrant relationships with every person.

Singing praise and worship songs during our evening visits had become a habit. Elizabeth really liked it. She always asked us to sing in her room, if we didn't initiate it ourselves. We had no self-consciousness about it. We sang to God "for Elizabeth". Sometimes she mouthed words in silence as we sang. Singing and focusing on Jesus to encourage Elizabeth encouraged us, too.

Her nurse heard us singing that night.

"Your singing together reminds me of the movies," he said. "It makes me feel like crying."

After we finished singing for the night, we prayed for her current needs, said our round of "I love yous," and left her for another night in ICU.

CHAPTER ELEVEN

The Lord Finally Had Me Where He Wanted Me

"She looks great!" said her nurse the next morning. "She's beaten this! Her lungs are clearer!"

He'd been gone for a week, but he was rotating back in to care for Elizabeth. He was really excited.

That type of response became common whenever anyone on the medical staff had been away from her for a week or more. Their amazement when they saw her again was contagious.

Elizabeth's note-writing quickly improved and became helpful to everyone. She seemed to have fun writing a batch of family love notes.

"Hi Dad. I ♥ you. I ♥ Mom. I ♥ you 2, Maggie. I ♥ Sarah. I miss John."

We'd grown to love John, too. One way of getting to know your daughter's boyfriend is to go through a medical crisis like Elizabeth's together. Since we'd been spending so much time with John, we learned he was fun to be with. Whatever we did in Elizabeth's room, John joined in. We noticed he fit in well with our family. He treated Maggie and Sarah like they were his own sisters. He was a blessing.

That morning, Maggie felt an urge to write a poem entitled "A Poem About God."

> "As I sit in this room in the ICU, I can't help but think
> of your love, so good and true.
> Your strength has given us hope. It has made it
> somewhat easy to cope.
> When I look at her lying in her bed, I am reminded of
> what you said,
> That when we ask in prayer and believe, what we ask, we
> will receive!
> So we ask that you would heal her and keep her safe
> from all she may encounter.
> We know you will provide for all her needs. In you we
> will rejoice as she succeeds.
> Now, with every heartbeat your perfect plan will be
> complete.
> With every breath of air you prove that you are the
> healer, no one can compare!"

Near lunch that day, Maggie, Matt and I were in Elizabeth's room when her nurse came in with a message.

"Dr. Abergel called and told me to tell you '100%,'" he said. "I don't know what that means, but he said you'd know."

We knew it meant 100% chance of survival—way up from 40–50% weeks ago!

"He also said that he'll be back on Monday and will do his best to extubate her then," the nurse added.

"Could this really be coming together?" we wondered.

We tried not to be too excited, but it didn't work. The doctor's words definitely stirred us up.

When we weren't in Elizabeth's room, there never seemed to be a shortage of people to talk to. In the waiting room, strangers sharing the ICU experience with their loved ones would really want to talk at times. The place brought out the desire to share medical trials and tribulations. That afternoon a woman told me the story of how her husband had died in that hospital four years earlier. She shared more than I wanted to know.

Since Elizabeth's hospital stay had turned from days to weeks, I'd begun to experience a new form of exhaustion—social interaction overload. Going at it for over twelve hours a day anywhere I went began to affect me. Sometimes I felt completely talked out. I knew I needed to be alone and silent. At those times I'd try to find a way to disappear temporarily.

As that particular day progressed, I felt I was on the verge of getting sick. So I went home to get some physical and social rest. As I left the hospital, I felt like the movie star, Gretta Garbo.

"I vant to be alone!" she'd said passionately.

I did too! I desperately wanted to be invisible for a short time.

Most people had given up trying to call our house by then, because we were never there. So, I didn't think of unplugging the phone. I'd just fallen asleep when the phone rang. The caller wanted an update. I couldn't believe it! It just wasn't fair! After the phone call, I rested on the bed a little longer and hoped sleep would return. It didn't. My nap was over.

I was so extremely tired yet unable to get any rest. I felt like crying, but I was too tired to cry. Instead I complained to the Lord.

"Lord, I can't even get a nap," I whined. "There's nowhere I can go to get away from people. Somehow they always find me. How do I handle this?"

Since her last visit, Jeri, along with Nancy (another sister), and a couple of other friends had decided to buy Sarah's prom dress for us. Jeri had made arrangements to shop with Sarah and shopping day had come. Jeri arrived early that morning raring to hit the dress shops.

When Matt saw that Elizabeth was having a good morning, he suggested I go with them. John was also there for a visit, and the two men said they'd stay and keep Elizabeth company. God unexpectedly opened up a pleasant bubble of time for me to get away, and I was elated.

It was somewhat late in the prom dress shopping season in Camarillo, and I felt concerned we might not find much. At the first shop, Sarah tried on at least five or six beautiful gowns. They fit well and she looked gorgeous. But it wasn't until we looked in the third shop that Sarah tried on a couple of dresses that lit up her face. The hard part for her was choosing the color, but she finally made her decision. Sarah absolutely loved the dress, and Jeri and I were so excited for her. Sarah and I were full of gratitude.

The topper was that we finished shopping within two to three hours. Some high school girls take days or weeks to find a dress they like. God knew we didn't have that kind of time, and He saved us from that kind of difficulty. I was amazed, relieved, and thankful. We had a successful and enjoyable time. Our God, the great healer and life-sustainer also cares about prom dresses for teenage girls!

After we returned to the hospital, Sarah couldn't wait to model her dress for Elizabeth. She even stood on a chair so her older sister could also see the bottom part of the dress. Elizabeth loved it, too.

In our absence, Matt had delivered a piece of mail to Elizabeth sent by a friend with travel plans. A note inside informed her that she and her husband were going on a trip to Berlin, Germany, Elbe River Cruise and Prague. She planned to write Elizabeth's name in the book of people needing prayer in some beautiful cathedrals they'd visit. She wanted the whole world to pray and praise God for Elizabeth.

For days we'd seen increasingly eager anticipation for Elizabeth to get off the ventilator soon, so I began thinking of a way to celebrate the big day. While I was out one afternoon running a quick errand, I bought a card, a cute plastic "Congratulations" key chain, and a huge, pink Mylar balloon in the shape of a rose.

That night we gave John some alone time with Elizabeth. When he came back out to the waiting room, he was especially excited. As usual, the rest of us were tired and ready to leave. We all walked down the hall, and as we went John took a treasure out of his pocket and showed it to Sarah. Elizabeth had just given him a note.

"I ♥ you," it read.

"Doesn't ♥ mean love?" John asked.

"Yes, ♥ means love," said Sarah.

John wanted to make sure he'd received the right message. He warmed up quickly to Elizabeth's love notes! Wasn't there some country and western song somewhere entitled "Love Can Bloom In An ICU Room?"

The next morning, they began another series of stress tests—temporarily removing ventilator support from Elizabeth. She kept trying to go for longer periods of time. She persevered and gave it her all. Her first try for the day went for a full hour. When they put her back on ventilator support, she appeared worn out again. She needed time to recover.

Then, late in the afternoon, Elizabeth's heart rate went very high without any apparent cause. She wasn't exercising her lungs when it happened. The nurse notified the doctor on call, and he advised her of measures to take to get it down. Despite those, it kept climbing. They reminded us that the risk of a very high heart rate is a heart attack. Stabs of fear began again.

By early evening, the doctor arrived looking very concerned. He was told Elizabeth's heart rate was 180 and her fever was 101.3. He carefully began to check every possible cause for such a high heart rate.

So many difficulties had affected her body over the past four weeks, and it all started to become unreal to me. It was hard to conceive of the pain and suffering she experienced. I imagined a line of credit for poor health with each new problem charged to Elizabeth's account.

As I watched the medical team work so urgently on her, I was reminded that the living organs and blood of my daughter were being attacked, weakened, and compromised. The danger was real. We went back to the waiting room where we prayed and waited for an update. After we prayed, I felt God start to slice little chunks of fear off my heart. He replaced them with His peace.

Matt and I weren't in the waiting room long when Jeri and her sons, Luc and Sam, came to visit. We loved seeing supportive faces. We explained Elizabeth's current heart rate crisis to them. After we visited with them for a while, Elizabeth's nurse came out to report that her heart rate had begun to decline slowly from 180 to 158. She was improving slightly. I exhaled a sigh of relief.

All along, doctors had been telling us that setbacks were a part of her kind of illness. Even with that in mind, Matt and I never knew when a new problem or setback would go for a jugular and freeze one of us in fear.

Elizabeth's high heart rate got a tight grip on Matt. He felt extremely discouraged because she'd been making good progress. He shut down almost completely.

"What if her heart rate gets out of whack again and shoots up even higher?" he asked himself. "What is causing this? I want her to have a normal heart rate."

Dinner time drew near, so we decided to get some pizza. Matt walked quietly to the car with us. While we ate with Jeri, Luc, and Sam that night, we all had a good visit except Matt. He really didn't like the high heart rate! He was stuck there. He sat at the table as silent as a stone.

When he thought about Elizabeth's problem, his mind jumped back a few weeks to the time a teenage boy had been brought into ICU with a high heart rate of 200. The doctor had been real concerned about him and thought he might not make it. They didn't know if his problem was drug induced or from some other cause. He survived and was released from ICU within a couple of days, but the part of his story that Matt was hung up on was the potential for death.

"What if Elizabeth has a heart attack?" dominated his thoughts. "I don't want her to die. She could die this very minute!"

I kept encouraging him to snap out of it, but he didn't. The rest of us finished our meal.

Sometimes distractions helped us immensely. Luc, a big football player who doesn't look at all like the artistic type, brought some artwork to show us from a class he'd recently taken. The pizza place was dimly lit, but we sat so close to Luc, we could see perfectly. We said "ooooo" and "awe" as he displayed each lovely piece.

"I got a good grade on my final with this next one," Luc said.

He showed us a rendition of an emblem from a fast food restaurant in California that doesn't exist in Nebraska where he'd attended college.

When his brief "art show in a pizza place" ended, Luc's mom, Jeri, sat back in her chair and smiled proudly. The only person who didn't find it a nice distraction was Matt.

When we returned to ICU, we received a full update on Elizabeth. We were relieved when the doctor told us an EKG indicated nothing was wrong with her heart other than the fast rate. He felt little changes were big things for Elizabeth. They'd exercised her lungs a lot that day, and the doctor's theory was that the exercising could have caused the higher heart rate. However, they also found the Pseudomonas bug in her sputum again.

"Oh no!" I moaned inwardly. "Not again!"

She'd been on a complicated antibiotic regimen already, but they changed the antibiotics quite a bit to handle the second round of infection.

By the next morning, Elizabeth had stabilized. Her new heart rate goal was to stay close to 120 and go no higher. Ventilator work stopped that day because she was sick and tired. Her body wasn't up for it. Her main job for the day was to rest. It was difficult to hear that, since they'd been so excited about getting her off the ventilator a few days earlier. God rejected our plans and timing. He slowed everything down again. We had to abandon intense desires for progress and do nothing. I discovered doing nothing was hard work.

Being forced to accept the "doing nothing" mode again gave me more time to think. I tried to be calm, but I felt like screaming.

"No!" I said to myself. "I can't sit here anymore watching Elizabeth get nowhere!"

I started talking to God, arguing my case over the answers to prayer He'd just sent.

"Lord, we prayed for You to prevent more hospital-acquired diseases," I told Him. "We prayed for You to help her progress off the ventilator, but You've allowed the opposite. I just don't get it!"

My Bible reminded me not to doubt that God knew what He was doing. I wanted to fully trust Him, to sit quietly knowing Elizabeth and all of us were securely in His hands, but I didn't feel that way.

Throughout our journey, God had to patiently teach me the same lessons over and over. I'm like many of His children who aren't always the sharpest or most cooperative of students. With us slow learners, God employs the repetition factor. He works continually to rewire thinking and teach His ways, which is no small task. Repetition is one of His persevering power tools.

One lesson I had great difficulty learning during our journey was "Understanding God's Timing". I continued to struggle with it. The Lord must have looked down on me tirelessly like a patient parent does when they answer their child's repeated questions on a long road trip—"Are we there yet? Are we there yet?"

I'd already asked "How long, O Lord?" so many times, I lost track.

Since God is eternal and He exists outside of our time constraints, we aren't always in tune with His timing. He has no human timepiece, yet He's never late. He fulfills His plans in perfect timing, known only to Him.

While He lived on earth, Jesus once taught Mary and Martha, sisters of a man named Lazarus, about His timing. Their story is recorded in John 11:1–45. They were close friends of Jesus. He loved them and had fellowship in their home often. They were a teachable family with a solid faith in Jesus.

Jesus happened to be gone with His disciples when Lazarus became very sick. The sisters sent word to Him to come help, because they knew He'd healed many others. But Jesus knew each purpose He planned to fulfill in the lives of all the people in the story. One purpose was to glorify God through the situation. Jesus also wanted more people to believe in Him.

However, people have a hard time thinking about God's glory or the spiritual condition of others around them when one of their loved ones is dying. Nevertheless, Jesus demonstrated "God time" by waiting two more days until His friend, Lazarus, had died before He went to him.

Great confusion hit both Martha and Mary about the timing of Jesus' arrival after they'd asked for His help. Lazarus had been in the tomb four days when He came to their home. Both women immediately made the same comment to Jesus when they spoke to Him individually.

"Lord, if you had been here, my brother would not have died."

They knew what He could do and they knew He loved them and their brother. Why did Jesus let Lazarus die?

Jesus was about to fulfill other plans that no one could envision. He'd teach Martha and those who'd study the story in John 11 through all generations about resurrection. He would perform a miracle and raise Lazarus back to life. The disciples would learn more of who Jesus was and many Jews who witnessed the miracle would begin to believe in Him.

He also knew some would not believe. Instead they'd report His actions to the Pharisees who would meet to devise plans to kill Him. All these things were in His plan. He allowed the proper amount of time for each of His purposes to take place. It was genius. Jesus had so much more in His plans than just healing his sick friend, Lazarus.

In Elizabeth's illness, Jesus was at work increasing our perseverance and trust. He seems to love stretching His people almost to the breaking point, even though He knows it can hurt so much. During indefinite periods of waiting, He was also teaching the massive prayer team He'd assembled on her behalf what persistent prayer was all about.

God's desire for me was to "be still, and know that I am God" (Psalm 46:10). I needed to trust Him—no questions asked. He was at work in ways I couldn't fathom, answering my earlier "whatever it takes" prayers.

⁓⦿⁓

I thought back to Day 1 when Elizabeth's situation first became life-threatening. The Lord did so many amazing things in our hearts. One much-needed position shift in my heart in regards to my marriage was done quietly behind-the-scenes. I was totally unaware of it until much later.

For years I'd made many self-reliant efforts to make my Christian marriage what I thought God wanted it to be. Whenever I entertained the thought that my husband wasn't interested in the things that mattered most to me, I took leadership and became very pushy.

One example of this was the time I heard about a popular six-week marriage seminar coming to our town. I really wanted to go and I asked Matt to go with me. He was resistant but I was persistent. Somehow we got there, but I quickly realized all I'd really done was drag him there each week. Sadly, neither of us got much from the seminar. Internally we butted heads over it. We lacked loving, respectful and teachable attitudes, so the Holy Spirit couldn't work.

I'd also become particularly skilled with one fleshly method where I pointed out parts of sermons Matt should apply to his life as we drove home from church. Actually, I demonstrated a critical spirit quite often.

Once I even criticized the time of day he chose to read his Bible. He read it at bedtime, and I was just sure that didn't give him time to think about what he'd read and apply it. I thought he'd fall asleep and immediately forget what he'd read. Can you say "legalistic?" My negative comments were never well-received. After a while, even positive comments were looked at with suspicion. It was hard for me to accept our inability to talk about the Lord together.

I also tried to function in my marriage with a broken forgiveness mechanism. I held stern conditions within me that determined whether or not I'd forgive Matt. If he came to me and apologized, I wouldn't forgive him if I felt he wasn't sincere or if I wasn't sure he wouldn't do it again.

For many years I failed to exercise the faith needed to forgive. I didn't understand Jesus' command to forgive a repentant person from my heart up to 490 times, even if it was for the same thing.

We'd had another spiritual problem for many years, without realizing it. We'd both had incorrect spiritual expectations of one another. This may have developed partly because we didn't understand or accept the way the Lord worked through our different spiritual gifts.

The Lord gave Matt the gift of helps, and He gave me the gift of teaching. As a teacher, I always wanted to dig deeper, study hard, and share a lot. But Matt was more affected by brief times in the Word, which then motivated him to get busy helping wherever he saw needs. Without knowing it, I put great pressure on Matt to be more like me, and he dug in his heels in resistance. It seemed like one of us always expected too much and the other expected too little.

I knew the scripture that reminded wives that a husband could be won without a word if the wife behaved in chaste, respectful ways, but I couldn't figure out how to become wordless. As a verbal and expressive person, I felt I should be free to say what I wanted whenever and however I wanted. I was so wrong. One politician recently said it wasn't wise to do the same things over and over and expect different results. That's what I'd been doing. My ineffective ways didn't increase the godliness of my marriage, no matter how many times I tried them.

In my own strength, my own natural attitudes and actions thwarted the progress I pursued, creating anger, frustration, and despair.

Back in Elizabeth's room, while I continued the work of doing nothing, Psalm 46:10 crossed my mind again and I thought about the opening phrase—"be still." I remembered this verse from the NASB version where the phrase "cease striving" is used. When I thought about the word striving, it sounded like what I'd been doing for a long time with my husband. The definition of strive is "to try hard, work hard, to struggle with, fight against, contend, or battle."

A couple of times in the past, I'd reached out to a godly woman to teach me how to be a godly wife. God began to use those times to make big progress, but, again, I was not the most teachable or persevering subject.

As I'd grown in my faith, I had true spiritual joy in my life, but the destructive effect of spiritual pride occasionally crept in. When I was most full of myself as a spiritual leader, I not only tried to lead Matt, I tried to lead God, too.

When God was at work, it remained difficult for me to be quiet and to figure out how to stay out of His way. I even found myself striving over how to cease striving.

Stay over there quietly and let me work, God would tell me.

After a short time, I'd move close to Him again.

"But what if I just..." I'd say.

He'd kindly interrupt my suggestion.

No, I'll handle it. I know what to do, He'd say.

I'd go back to sitting quietly, but a little later, I'd return and try to force my way in again.

"Maybe it would be good if I said..." I'd say urgently.

Then He'd lovingly shush me and go about His work.

During those times, the Lord stopped some of my striving and began to put me into trust mode with my marriage. Some progress was made. As the godly Christian women discipled and ministered to me, each was very encouraging, but in our time together, obstacles toward lasting change seemed to keep coming. Sometimes my own emotional pain and depression slowed improvement efforts.

Not long after we stopped meeting together, my sly sin nature would passionately start trying to make something happen again.

I wouldn't stop interrupting the Lord and trying to change His plans and His perfect ways, so His work became shelved for a time. I consistently failed to understand that my ways to be a wife were not automatically His ways just because I was a believer. I kept messing with His equipment too often and tried to substitute my power for His. God knew extreme measures would be required in His next dealings with me.

Just before Elizabeth got sick, when I prayed, "whatever it takes," He knew I was finally ready to be still and *stay out of His way,* but He was sure it would be no small thing to achieve. He knows me all too well. It would take His miracle power. He had to "lift me up, move me, and keep me out of His way" Himself. On Elizabeth's first critical day, He did that. He finally had me where He wanted me. He used severe adversity to put me in that proper place.

Elizabeth's crisis required all the time and energy I had each day. I had none left to use toward our marriage in any way. I didn't even give working on my marriage one thought. What a restful place! "Being still" the way God wanted was wonderful! At last, He had glorious freedom to work unhindered.

God knows and loves each of His children so well. If He could create well-being and spiritual maturity in them with the slightest promptings, He'd surely do that. But we are resisters. Our bullish sinful natures can fight Him for control at every turn. Every human heart can become hard, obstinate, rebellious, blind, and deaf.

Our journey was teaching me that sometimes He must use the toughest things to break us, to make our hearts pliable, soft, moldable to His touch, and to unstop our ears so we hear His voice. God knows that sometimes His work will require His big guns—suffering, crisis, and calamity, or even a series of these. His use of pain, suffering, and timing is masterful. He is the only true spiritual healer. He knows what will work and how much pressure, pain, and hardship is necessary in individual lives to break up spiritual maladies ranging from rejection and apathy all the way to pride.

He knows the perfect measure of "whatever it takes" for each person He's created. And He knows how to use His superior and unusual ways of doing things to transform lives so He can use them in His kingdom work.

From a human perspective, going through suffering may seem like a mistake. God may appear cruel. But at times He must show His love by correcting His child and preventing deeper suffering that would result if He allowed further progress in a harmful direction. From His perspective, God knows suffering actually moves us along toward our own ultimate goals.

As I wanted to resist facing another setback for Elizabeth that day, He hadn't given me the right to end the suffering at that point in her recovery, even though I desperately wanted to. My vision and perspective were very limited, and my own timing was selfish. If He had allowed me to end our struggle when I thought best, much of His work wouldn't have been completed in the time He'd chosen to do it.

After a while, the Lord brought some composure to me. I sat near Elizabeth's bed as His wisdom took its place in my mind. I remembered that I hadn't added a heart of surrender to my most recent prayers. The outcome may have been the same had I also prayed, "Not my will but Thine be done," but my heart would have been peaceful.

Gradually the Lord showed me what "doing nothing" really entailed—watch her rest and keep praying. I knew, again, that was the only thing I could do. I thought about key words in her update that morning—stop and rest. And I considered one of God's key words—trust. Words like stop, rest, and trust seemed like such slow words. They can't be hurried. The Lord carefully guided me to a place where I looked at that day with His perspective.

I use hours like these to grow and mature My people, He said.

CHAPTER TWELVE

Dance

AFTER ELIZABETH'S SETBACK THE PREVIOUS night, the doctors considered the possibility that her recovery might take longer than they'd been thinking. They'd hoped to permanently remove her current IV line soon. Instead, they needed to change it.

Earlier, a PIC Line had been discussed. It was an upgrade from the IV lines she'd been using. It would make administering vital fluids and medications much easier. It could also stay in one place for up to three weeks without worry of infection. Her doctor decided the time had come to have the PIC Line procedure done.

Elizabeth was stable, so they scheduled it for that afternoon. They planned to wheel her bed across the hall to radiology for the procedure. By the time they were ready, Sarah was done with school for the day and she'd joined Maggie and me at the hospital. Before they took Elizabeth, we prayed by her bed for it to go well.

We were told they'd bring her out a certain door. It would be the first time she left ICU in over a month. We waited nearby and kept our eyes on that door. We wanted to wave at her and look supportive so she wouldn't become anxious.

Just before it was time to go, her nurse unhooked her from the power sources in her room and began using a portable ventilator, a hand-held bag that was squeezed at regular intervals to supply oxygen.

Suddenly, the wheels of her bed began moving. The ICU door opened. Her bed was surrounded by nurses, a respiratory therapist, and the radiologist. They wheeled her down the hall next to the window. She could see the sky, sunshine, and tree tops through the windows.

Maggie, Sarah, and I waved, smiled, and called to her, and as she and her entourage approached, she looked at us and gave us her raised eyebrow look. She even slightly raised her hand at the wrist to return a small wave. The medical staff continued carefully wheeling her bed and encouraging her all along the way.

As she passed us, we called out to her.

"You'll be fine, Elizabeth!"

Our voices trailed off as the radiology doors opened, received her and her bed, and then quietly eased shut.

The PIC Line procedure went well and she was returned to her ICU room and re-connected to all the important tubes, plugs, and medications. Once she was settled into her room again, she and her sisters watched some Disney movies using a TV and VCR unit a nurse had brought in recently. Elizabeth enjoyed that little luxury so much that she and Maggie made a list of movies to retrieve from home or the video rental place for her hospital viewing pleasure.

⁂

Later that afternoon, I met a woman in the waiting room whose husband had been diagnosed with Escherichia coli, or E. coli, infection. Before I heard all the details of his situation, fear immediately surged into me.

"Isn't that potentially deadly?" I asked myself. "Why is this man back in ICU somewhere near Elizabeth? What if the E. coli infection spreads to her, too?"

Fear bullied me again. Without all the facts, it manufactured pressures and twisted reality. I'd discovered that fear so often made things seem much worse than they actually were. As I listened to the woman explain, I found out the E. coli was contained in her husband's intestines, so he wasn't contagious.

I told her I'd pray for her husband, but I struggled with selfish motives as I prayed.

"The sooner he gets better and goes home, the sooner thoughts of E. coli will stop tormenting my own mind," I thought.

Even with clarifying information, fear kept trying to work me over.

As that slow day drew to a close, I thought back to Elizabeth's brief hall ride. It was exciting seeing her somewhere other than her ICU room. We couldn't wait for the day we'd see her somewhere other than the hospital.

※

Dr. Abergel returned to care for Elizabeth two days later. We'd missed him and were thrilled he was back. He felt optimistic about her extubation. She'd improved enough from her recent high heart rate episode and illness for him to start more stress tests. That day she temporarily breathed off the ventilator for even longer periods than before. Her longest time was a two-hour session. Exhaustion, again, accompanied her return to ventilator support.

The doctors had been watching for the right time to try to extubate Elizabeth.

"Will it happen when they hope?" we wondered. "Will she be able to stay off the ventilator? Or will she feel forced to try to do what she knows she can't do?"

We weren't sure they'd try to remove the ventilator the following day, but John told us he wanted to be there. He knew it would be a huge event in her recovery. So he drove in, ready to share in the celebration if and when it happened. Elizabeth would be the first to tell you it was always good to see John.

Meanwhile, back in Sarah's high school life, she kept up with the swim team. I was glad she still had normal activities to keep her busy. That afternoon she had a swim meet, and I left the hospital to see her final races. I loved watching her swim. As I thought about my two healthy daughters, I sometimes worried that the hospital life we were living was too much for them. They were young. And they were so unselfish with their time. But they both persevered in their tireless support and prayer for the sister they loved so dearly.

※

Upon arriving in ICU the next morning, we saw Dr. Abergel in decision-making mode.

"Is this the day to try extubation?" he'd been asking himself. "Is Elizabeth ready?"

Elizabeth looked worn out from breathing work the previous day, and her nurse told us she hadn't slept well the night before.

"Elizabeth, do you feel ready to get off the ventilator?" I asked.

"No," she replied.

When we talked to Dr. Abergel, we told him what Elizabeth had said. He took that into account. Then he explained his perspective.

"I feel today provides the best window of opportunity she's going to get," he said. "We've been waiting for her to be well and strong enough to do it. I'm not fully confident it will be successful, but I'll give it a 60% chance of success. She deserves a chance to try."

He eventually decided to go forward with his plan to extubate her. Shortly after noon, Dr. Abergel went into Elizabeth's room and spoke with her. He started by telling her she'd been in the hospital for over a month. Then he explained what they were about to do. Even though she wasn't sure she could do it, she was willing to try.

The believers were praying. At 12:25, the doctor took Elizabeth off the ventilator. *Praise God!*

Not long after he took the tube out, Dr. Abergel spoke with us.

"I don't think she would have done this well without your praying. It went so smoothly."

It was looking good. We were ecstatic. We made update phone calls and stayed around the ICU waiting room in case anything came up. A while later, Dr. Abergel took us into Elizabeth's room so we could see how she was doing. She was inhaling an oxygen mist over her mouth, and she appeared to be working a little hard to breathe. We all tried to remain optimistic. We left to grab a bite to eat while Matt returned to work.

The mood to celebrate big time came over us. The large, pink Mylar balloon in the shape of a rose I'd bought to celebrate earlier was deflated and lying on the floor at home. I took it to the store and had more helium put into it. John and Maggie ran errands of their own while I was out. Sarah stayed home and did homework.

Before we got back, Elizabeth's nurse called our house. I just happened to return home at the same time Maggie and John drove up. When we went in the house, Sarah started to give us the message.

"Elizabeth's nurse called…"

That was all she had to say. A sense of dread came over us immediately. We all sat down to hear Sarah finish the message.

"Elizabeth began having difficulty and they had to reintubate her."

Once we heard that, we sat in our living room in silence for a long time. We were speechless. Our minds unsuccessfully tried to understand what happened.

After a while, we remembered our role as Elizabeth's encouragement team, so we quickly got ready and went to be with her. We knew she'd feel discouraged.

When we entered ICU, Dr. Abergel looked very sad. Actually, we all did. The doctor briefly explained the problem.

"She was inhaling okay, but she wasn't able to exhale enough carbon dioxide," he said. "Her body just couldn't do some of the things we were asking of it."

Elizabeth's nurse that week had an unusually compassionate face. We approached him outside her room.

"I'm sorry," he said tenderly.

"Thank you," I said.

When we entered her room, Elizabeth's disappointment was heartbreaking to see. She was so discouraged. Maggie, Sarah, John, and I tried to comfort her. I got close to her face and sort of hugged her.

"I'm so sorry!" I said.

Elizabeth and I cried together. I knew she'd tried extremely hard.

"We'll just figure out what to do next," I said.

I looked up and saw John gently shaking his head in a "No, don't do that" motion. Suddenly, I realized I was breaking the "don't upset the patient" rule. I stopped crying as quickly as I could. Then we all stayed near Elizabeth and gave her loads of love and support.

Later when we were walking out of ICU to get dinner, Dr. Abergel stopped us to talk. My heart was broken. I was struggling to process the fact that she couldn't get off the machine, and I was fearful about her future. I shared my tearful thoughts with Dr. Abergel.

"Here's my deepest unspoken fear—I'm afraid Elizabeth will never be able to get off the ventilator."

It felt good for a brief moment to be honest. I didn't have to put on a brave, cheerful face with Dr. Abergel.

"What happens to people who can't get off a ventilator?" I asked.

"There are facilities for respirator-dependent people," he said. "I recommend one in Los Angeles. They have the best reputation for getting tough case patients off ventilators."

That gave me a little hope.

We wanted Elizabeth off the ventilator so badly. She wanted it, too. Sometimes when people have intense desires like that, I've noticed we create a false optimism from our own emotions. We stir up our own excitement and tell ourselves, "If I think enough positive thoughts, I can make something happen." I think we feel more tempted to create false optimism whenever God says "no" or "wait" in answer to our prayers.

That optimism exerts a form of pressure or manipulation. We don't like giving up our plans, so we forcefully try "ramming a square object into a round hole." We want our own way, and when we refuse to hold our plans loosely, we tend to become dictators. If it keeps going, we can aggressively pull others into it with us. We may even try to shame them if they don't want to join us.

The problem with false optimism is that the thinking and activity are based on self. Someone has a series of self-reliant thoughts like:

"I'm in charge. I'm calling the shots. I have the power to make things happen."

There isn't any strong foundation underneath those thoughts. Maybe there isn't even much truth present in the false optimism.

In the prophet Jeremiah's day, false optimism was a big problem. God told Jeremiah to start working on getting rid of it.

> "Yes, this is what the Lord Almighty, the God of Israel, says: 'Do not let the prophets and diviners among you deceive you. Do not listen to the dreams you encourage them to have. They are prophesying lies to you in my name. I have not sent them,' declares the Lord" (Jeremiah 29:8–9).

Earlier in the same book, God speaks to Jeremiah about messages He has not given.

> "This is what the Lord Almighty says: 'Do not listen to what the prophets are prophesying to you; they fill you with false hopes. They speak visions from their own minds, not from the mouth of the Lord. They keep saying to those who despise me, "The Lord says: You will have peace." And to all who follow the stubbornness of their hearts they say, "No harm will come to you." But which of them has stood in the council of the Lord to see or to hear His word?'" (Jeremiah 23:16–18).

It appears God wanted to develop and sharpen the discernment of His people. In every generation, He never wanted them forgetting He was their God. They were to depend on Him, not themselves. God tells us to check with Him before we make plans.

> "Now listen, you who say, 'Today or tomorrow we will go to this or that city, spend a year there, carry on business and make money.' Why, you do not even know what will happen tomorrow. What is your life? You are a mist that appears for a little while and then vanishes. Instead, you ought to say, 'If it is the Lord's will, we will live and do this or that.' As it is you boast and brag. All such boasting is evil" (James 4:13–16).

When a plan based on false optimism doesn't turn out the way we hope, the crash and burn can be painful. It may leave us greatly disillusioned. God has always wanted us to sidestep these crashes and follow His expert leading. Keeping our hearts surrendered to Him helps.

God encourages us not to fully trust our own understanding.

> "Trust in the Lord with all your heart and lean not on your own understanding; in all your ways acknowledge Him, and He will make your paths straight" (Proverbs 3:5–6).

The apostle Paul demonstrated the same principle when he made plans with the Philippians. He shows us God-dependent thinking and planning.

"I hope in the Lord Jesus to send Timothy to you soon, that I also may be cheered when I receive news about you" (Philippians 2:19).

Since our desires for Elizabeth's full recovery were intense, we needed to learn that there was a fine line between reliances. At any given time, we were fully relying either on God, self, or others. Only God-reliance kept us on the right path. When I rely on God, He prevents me from crossing over the fine line into another falsely optimistic reliance.

My battle was against my selfish inclination to believe that I knew it all. For instance, one piece of truth came from Elizabeth's doctors consistently.

"Setbacks are a part of her kind of illness."

But, at times my false optimism system would automatically reject that truth without even considering it. It was true, but I didn't want to believe it. I stubbornly insisted on hearing only statements that supported what I wanted. To be discerning and wise requires I seek God to discover what is true. It means I listen to everything and listen for His clear guidance. Then I am to stand firm in the position He's led me to. Confusion will always reign when I refuse to do this.

The whole family plus John went into Elizabeth's room together for the after-dinner visit that night. Right when we got there, she wrote a note.

"Sing."

With hearts full of pain and uncertainty, we started right in singing worship and praise songs. It helped all of us to refocus on God again. We each had the same desperate need for God's help to continue on our journey. We knew there weren't answers to our stabbing questions and fears. So we let God, in His beauty, push them out of our minds yet again. We found our joy and hope in Him alone.

After a severe climbing mishap in the Sierras and living for years with continual, insistent pain, author and speaker Tim Hansel learned about finding joy in every circumstance. It's the same joy Elizabeth discovered and shared with us that night.

In his book, *You Gotta Keep Dancin'*, he shared his thoughts about the time he discovered a powerful scripture verse—"The joy of the Lord is my strength" (Nehemiah 8:10).

> "God reminded me again and again that I cannot choose to be strong, but I can choose to be joyful," he said. "And when I'm willing to do that, strength will follow...If we are to have this kind of joy in our lives, we must first discover what it looks like. It is not a feeling; it is a *choice*. It is not based upon circumstances; it is based upon attitude. It is free, but it is not cheap. It is the by-product of a growing relationship with Jesus Christ. It is a promise, not a deal. It is available to us when we make ourselves available to him. It is something that we can receive by invitation and by choice. It requires commitment, courage, and endurance."

He came to the following conclusion:

> "The will of God for me was to 'be joyful always; pray continually; and give thanks in all circumstances.' 1 Thessalonians 5:16–18. Otherwise I am in danger of quenching the Spirit."[10]

That night, Elizabeth, like Tim Hansel, was determined not to be guilty of "putting off joy until [her] circumstances improved."

We continued our singing in Elizabeth's room. One chorus we sang spoke of God's ability to make all things beautiful in His perfect timing. Another reminded us of the peace and comfort that come when we cast our burdens at Jesus' feet.

We also read a couple of Bible verses that came to mind.

> "Brothers, as an example of patience in the face of suffering, take the prophets who spoke in the name of the Lord. As you know, we consider blessed those who have

---

10   Tim Hansel, You Gotta KeepDancin' © 1985 (Life Journey: Colorado Springs, Colorado) #47, 54-55.

persevered. You have heard of Job's perseverance and have seen what the Lord finally brought about. The Lord is full of compassion and mercy" (James 5:10–11).

As we finished our praise time, we were full of God's joy and strength. We could tell the Lord had entered Elizabeth's ICU room in a special way and filled our hearts to the brim. We kept learning that when we stood firm in God-reliance, we focused on His abilities to do anything He chose. Those things that seemed impossible for us were simple for Him. Our optimism and confidence were to be in Him alone.

Later during our visit, Elizabeth asked her dad to dance. In our many hours in Elizabeth's room, we did anything and everything that lightened the mood or distracted her from pain and anxiety. Elizabeth, Maggie, Sarah, and I watched as Matt became a different person through his daughter's illness. In the past, his daughters had a hard time convincing him to be silly. It was such a change when we saw a serious, practical, quiet man become fun and goofy without any hesitation. He did some of the weirdest things to make Elizabeth smile or laugh. He wasn't much of a dancer, but we saw him "dance" for Elizabeth.

We left John alone with Elizabeth to say goodnight. When he was ready to leave, he came out to the waiting room with a note from Elizabeth, which I read out loud.

"Today's one month since I've been in the hospital. I can't wait to talk to the nurses and staff. They've seen God's amazing work time and time again and my friends and family have been a great witness, too."

After I read the note, I looked up. John and Matt had tears in their eyes.

CHAPTER THIRTEEN

From Bad to Worse

Dr. Abergel was at the desk in front of Elizabeth's room when Maggie and I arrived the next morning. He was busy making lots of phone calls, so we went to visit with Elizabeth. When she'd been unable to stay off the ventilator, it got all the collaborating doctors on the same page. That morning, new plans were in the works.

When he had some free moments, Dr. Abergel called me to the desk to update me.

"We're not seeing a significant amount of improvement," he said.

He also reported a new concern about the unknown extent of scarring, or fibrosis, in her lungs. If there was a large amount of scarring, the ultimate treatment was a lung transplant. Dr. Abergel felt they needed to make drastic changes that day.

Tides of fear began to surge into me again. The Lord shot a verse to my mind.

"You will keep in perfect peace him whose mind is steadfast, because he trusts in You" (Isaiah 26:3).

I needed that as I faced another day full of rapid-fire, "pray-as-you-go-through-it" challenges.

One of the other doctors on Elizabeth's team was a well-known cardiovascular thoracic surgeon at St. John's Regional Medical Center in Oxnard. He feared it was possible the team was missing something important.

After considering all the input and finalizing his decisions, Dr. Abergel made four important recommendations. First, he prescribed doing a tracheotomy. He explained that it would make Elizabeth much more comfortable and allow them to go more slowly as they worked to progress her off the ventilator.

Next, Dr. Abergel suggested doing the open-lung biopsy they'd wanted to do earlier. During that surgery, they would open the chest wall, take a lung sample and send it to the laboratory to be analyzed by a microbiologist. They could finally have a good look at what was in her lungs. The infectious disease doctor was still highly in favor of it.

Since St. John's Regional Medical Center in Oxnard was a facility that was better suited for the open-lung biopsy, Dr. Abergel recommended transferring Elizabeth there. He felt the transfer really needed to be done. The Oxnard facility was a bigger hospital with more resources, and all of the doctors involved in her case rotated through there much of the time. He also wanted us to hear from each of them, including the thoracic surgeon.

Lastly, he said they felt they weren't getting an accurate picture of what was going on in her lungs from the x-rays, so he wanted a CAT scan or CT scan done of her lungs. This would provide a three-dimensional view with more information than a two-dimensional x-ray.

Matt and I eventually consented to the doctor's recommendations. So they made plans to perform the two procedures the following day in an operating room in the Oxnard hospital.

Next, Dr. Abergel took care of numerous details to arrange the transfer. As he spoke to the people preparing an ICU bed for Elizabeth at the new hospital, I heard him end the conversation with an additional order.

"Elizabeth is a very special patient. I want you to take very good care of her."

While these plans were in the works, Nancy was driving up from Huntington Beach to visit Elizabeth and take Maggie and me to lunch that day. Nancy is a strong woman, always full of faith. She's very skilled at building others up. All my daughters knew Nancy's sense of humor was a great pick me up. In her own life, she's victoriously dealt with a couple of very difficult health issues through the years. It was great to see her deliver a brand new batch of kindness and love to Elizabeth.

Even after such a great time in the Lord the night before, the reality of the failed extubation had crashed in on Elizabeth that morning with fresh despair. When Nancy looked into her eyes, she saw her deep disappointment.

"It looks like Elizabeth has given up hope," said Nancy during lunch.

Maggie and I agreed. The extubation failure took Elizabeth quite low that day.

After Nancy left, Maggie and I prepared to vacate Elizabeth's ICU room. Her wall had been covered with cards, pictures, and notes. We packed everything up that had been part of her "home" for the last month.

Elizabeth wanted to say thank you and goodbye to familiar, favorite nurses, but they weren't there that day. However, several respiratory and physical therapists who'd worked with her stopped by to give encouraging send-offs.

By mid afternoon transport people arrived, and the ambulance pulled up to the ER entrance. We checked on Elizabeth once more, prayed for a safe trip, and then left her in ICU. While waiting in the hall, I wrote a brief update and placed it on the table in the ICU waiting room so people would know where Elizabeth had gone.

At last, they were ready to go. The ICU door opened and Elizabeth was wheeled out. We waved and smiled. Once they got to the ambulance, it took them a while to get her situated inside. She was surrounded by everything that was needed to get her to the new hospital safely.

Maggie and I walked to one car while Matt and Sarah got into another. Finally, we saw the ambulance pulling into the street. Suddenly, the siren turned on. Maggie and I watched it speed away.

On the road in a big city, we'd seen ambulances drive by quite often. That day it impressed us quite differently since the one inside was my daughter and Maggie's sister. As we started to make the twenty-minute drive, Maggie began to cry. We rode the rest of the way in silence.

When we arrived at the new hospital, they were getting Elizabeth out of the ambulance and taking her back into the hospital. Just the sight of it delivered a punch to my own heart.

"My daughter is still extremely ill," I thought. "She needs more intensive care. My heart aches for her to be well again."

Not long after we began our drive to St. John's Regional Medical Center in Oxnard, Tami walked down the hall in the Camarillo hospital toward the waiting room.

That day, as she got near the room, she noticed it was dark and we weren't there.

"Oh, Lord…" she thought.

I was so glad I left a note explaining where Elizabeth went. I wanted to avoid the dread of her sudden absence with no information for her prayer supporters. That would have been cruel.

Matt, Maggie, Sarah and I were told how to find the combined ICU/CCU (Coronary Care Unit) waiting room on the second floor. The new waiting room was so different. It was noisy and full of people of various ages. There was a large soft drink machine in one corner that had a loud, continual hum. The room was bigger and instead of chairs, there were lots of couches.

On one couch, I saw an elderly woman sitting next to two adult women—probably her daughters. Their faces looked weary and their eyes were red. A chaplain sitting on a nearby couch leaned toward them slightly. After he spoke gently to them, they appeared grief-stricken. Later I noticed they'd all left the room.

There were also a couple of tables with chairs in one corner. A woman was sitting at one table thumbing nonchalantly through a magazine. A high school student sat at the other looking at a math book.

One man sat alone in the corner of another couch across the room. He had a pained expression on his face. I imagined thoughts of his loved one suffering great pain dominating his thoughts.

Extraordinary things seemed to be going on in the lives of the people there.

It was also a busy room. People were going in and out a lot. I thought it would have been quite difficult to pray in a room like that the way we had in Camarillo.

At the new hospital, the ICU and CCU doors were kept locked, so if a visitor wanted to get inside, a buzzer had to be pushed by the medical staff inside to grant access. Only two people were allowed in a patient's room at one time. That would be a new challenge for us.

As they settled Elizabeth in her room, they hooked her up to a ventilator that was so new and advanced, many of the respiratory therapists weren't sure how to make it do all it could. At first glance, the ICU was huge and very modern-looking. There were more beds and a much larger desk area. Elizabeth's ICU room was larger too, and it even had a phone in it.

By early evening, the CAT scan of her lungs was completed. Our family had been waiting around for a while to hear the results. We gave up and decided to get some dinner.

Just as we began walking down the hall, one of Elizabeth's doctors walked up to us with another doctor we didn't know. The new doctor said "hi" and introduced himself as the thoracic surgeon in that hospital.

As it turns out, he was the doctor who came to St. John's Pleasant Valley Hospital in Camarillo and inserted two chest tubes into Elizabeth's lungs on Day 1.

He spoke to us with authority.

"We just looked at your daughter's CAT scan," he said. "There has been no improvement over time. Her lungs are completely destroyed. They are horrendous and terrible. I've never seen such lungs! They won't improve. It's really not looking good."

The four of us were totally shocked. He used such horrid words! But he wasn't done.

"You should start looking into lung transplantation," he went on. "USC and Cedars-Sinai would be good to talk to about transplants."

"How long do lung transplants last?" Matt asked.

"I'm not sure," he said.

"Transplants are not done frequently," he continued. "Possibly they could do transplants within a couple of days to months. The results are actually pretty good."

"Elizabeth has multiple air pockets within her lungs," he added. "The influenza started the whole process over and over. Her lungs are completely scarred."

When he saw so much lung damage in the CAT scan report, he decided against doing the open-lung biopsy.

"What's the use?" he asked himself.

He concluded his report by telling us that the tracheotomy the following day would make her more comfortable. He also felt she was in reasonably stable condition.

Before he left, he asked if we wanted to go in and report the new findings to Elizabeth.

After a stunned pause, Matt spoke up.

"We'll wait," he said, sensing we needed time to think.

The doctors left.

We felt like a bomb had gone off inside of us. Everything went numb in an instant. We were blasted almost back to the beginning of Elizabeth's illness. The wind was knocked out of us and we could barely breathe. Our bodies were almost too weak to stand or walk. We felt shaky and insecure.

At that moment, the main thing the four of us knew was that we wanted to get out of there. We left the hospital in silence. We walked like zombies to our car and got inside. Then we sat there speechless—for a very long time.

Even though our hearts and spirits felt crushed, Matt was trying to grab hold of truths he'd learned at the beginning of the journey.

"I have no control over this situation," he told himself, struggling to remember. "Elizabeth is in God's hands. He is in control of everything."

A while later, Matt drove us to a fast food place nearby for dinner. No one was hungry, but we went through the motions of eating. We chewed and swallowed dispassionately. At some point, we tried to start talking to each other again. None of us believed how hopeless things sounded!

The new doctor made it sound like there was no way her lungs would last and that she had a very slim chance again. We asked each other lots of questions.

"Does it sound like she's now way worse than at the beginning?" I asked.

"How could she be so close to extubation one day and in such desperate need of a transplant the next?" asked Matt.

"Is this doctor saying she'll die right away without a transplant?" asked Maggie.

No one thought that was the case, but we didn't know. We weren't able to understand.

"Lord, what will happen to Elizabeth?" I prayed silently. "I'm afraid for her future! What do we do now?"

Processing the new update was incredibly painful. None of us knew what to make of it. We wondered why the pulmonologists had such a different take on her condition. We asked ourselves why Dr. Abergel wasn't there. We sure wished he was!

We had a most pressing question to answer during dinner—'What should we tell Elizabeth tonight?'

"If we tell her when we go back, how will it affect her?" I wondered. "She's already quite discouraged."

We'd been carefully trained in Camarillo to keep bad news from her so she would keep a good, positive attitude. We decided to keep that up. We wouldn't tell her that night. We'd pray for God to let us know the right time to tell her. We felt we needed more time to figure out what we were supposed to do.

Before returning to the hospital that night, we planned what we would and wouldn't say.

"We'll have to do the best acting of our lives to make Elizabeth feel nothing is wrong," I said to Maggie and Sarah.

I knew it would be difficult, but we'd become a great team. As we returned to the hospital, we knew our mission. We were determined to show Elizabeth our love and support like always. We wouldn't reveal the burning, terrifying words we'd heard just an hour earlier.

However, the report continued to overwhelm us that night. We felt the need to inform everyone immediately instead of waiting for our regular morning update. But the thought of passing on that news filled us with frightful thoughts. The first person I called was Joy. She listened sympathetically and then prayed over the phone. I began to cry. Then we made many more calls. Each time we spoke about it, it felt terrible.

Between calls, since I saw no end to Elizabeth's troubles in sight, I realized something inside me had snapped. I was afraid the stressful hospital lifestyle would become permanent for us. In my exhaustion and pain, my faith started to weaken. I couldn't shake the feeling that we might have to start all over again, and I dreaded thinking about that. I was spent. A damaging thought began to work its way deep inside my heart and mind and attack my trust in God—'I absolutely can't take this anymore!'

The Holy Spirit was prompting me to receive God's wisdom, but I wasn't listening to Him too well that night. He wanted me to remember and understand.

You haven't made it this far in your own strength, He said. *You did it in the strength God gave you.*

Unknowingly, I allowed a small amount of spiritual hardness to affect my heart.

I despised the thought of passing the awful report on to John.

"No way!" said John when he heard it. "What does it mean? Will she be a vegetable? Will she be disabled? Can she recover?"

He felt afraid and confused.

This news hit all of us quite hard. After hearing about the transplant recommendation, John couldn't keep his mind on school work any longer. His mom requested a reprise for him from Biola. He'd take his finals a little later in the summer. He just needed to be with Elizabeth, and that was that.

We drove home and went to bed. God blessed us with a good night's sleep, and the next morning we were ready to get moving. Elizabeth was scheduled for the tracheotomy early that morning and Sarah's prom was that night. A very full day was lined up for us.

Having a little time to think about last night's CAT scan results and their delivery made me think of one word—brutal.

Shortly after we arrived in the waiting room, a couple of friends showed up. They came with hearts full of compassion, comfort, helpful suggestions, and fresh hope to share. Now when friends "stopped by," the hospital was out of their way.

"Matt and I are eager to talk to the doctor, so I'll have to leave shortly," I told them.

The three of us huddled together and prayed in the corner of the noisy waiting room. We could barely hear each other as we prayed. Before I left them, I shared my scattered thoughts for the day.

"Sarah's prom is tonight and I still have to iron her dress...Matt and I want to be home to take pictures and see her off...we don't want to leave Elizabeth alone this afternoon..."

Just then, Tami stopped me.

"I'll sit with Elizabeth," she said, ready to meet the need immediately.

"Are you sure?" I asked her. "Do you have time? That would help so much!"

She assured me she'd be happy to do it. That was a load off my mind. She planned to return before we left to be prom parents.

That morning, back at Biola University, John's band led in worship. The chapel organizers gave him time to report Elizabeth's new need, and then the body of believers there lifted her again before the throne of grace. After chapel, he drove out to be with Elizabeth. Again, God faithfully sent sufficient help for the day.

Since the previous night, Elizabeth's doctors had been busy talking to a lung specialist at Cedars-Sinai Medical Center in Los Angeles. Among other things, Cedars-Sinai was known to excel in lung transplantation work.

As we entered ICU, we immediately saw one doctor on the team sitting at the desk. We greeted him and he gave us his take on Elizabeth's condition.

"This is a little discouraging, but I think she still may get better," he said. "Every day she's progressing. The question is—is her improvement enough to support her need for oxygen? She still has a lot of disease in her lungs. I think a lot of what they saw on the CAT scan could be infection."

As our conversation ended, Matt and I told him we'd both be happy to donate one of our lungs to Elizabeth if they could use them.

"We all want what's best for Elizabeth," he responded as tears welled up in his eyes. "We want her to get better. There's only so much we can do. We're just people."

Elizabeth's tracheotomy had been performed successfully that morning, and we went in to see her after we talked to the doctor. She looked beautiful. We could see her teeth again, and her smile was lovely.

We were hoping she'd be able to talk, since she'd had over a month of silence, but she couldn't. For some reason, her surgeon had decided to put in the type of tube that didn't allow the patient to speak. We had to get over that disappointment. We focused on seeing her so much more comfortable. That was a thrilling, pleasant gift!

Dr. Abergel arrived a while later. We desperately wanted his input. We left Elizabeth's room and talked with him at the desk.

"Even though Elizabeth is close to her best from the time she came, a lot of things have developed," he said. "The CAT scan gave us a clearer picture of her lungs and it showed a lot of significant findings such as fibrosis, inflammation, and infection. We also saw that both lungs had lots of undesirable lung infiltrate, and that quite a bit of lung was collapsed."

These were all unfavorable lung words.

Dr. Abergel had also talked to the Cedars-Sinai lung specialist, who'd taken an interest in Elizabeth. He'd recommended more chest tube therapy to eradicate any air pockets, or pneumothorax.

"How many chest tubes should we use?" asked Dr. Abergel.

"As many as it takes," replied the lung specialist.

The specialist also said it sounded like Elizabeth was showing some improvement. He recommended giving her two to three weeks before they re-evaluated her. Then, only if there was no improvement, he told them, it would be good to transfer her to Cedars-Sinai for further evaluation. He also mentioned that patients had to be either a little better or severely worse than Elizabeth in order to get a lung transplant.

Since I'd been a close observer of Elizabeth's ventilator work, I made a request of Dr. Abergel.

"Can you have everyone go very, very slowly when trying to lower her ventilator settings?" I asked. "It seems like every time they make aggressive steps, she's unable to go where they want her to. I've seen them move one setting for pressure support down from 12 to 6. Can they move it from 12 to 11 or 10 instead? I really think the tiniest of steps may work better for Elizabeth's *slow* case. I don't want to see more failure and frustration for her."

"That's what we planned to do—starting today," he said.

Our crucial update drew to a close. Before we left him to rejoin Elizabeth, he shared a final comment.

"The thoracic surgeon feels Elizabeth needs a lung, but as her primary doctor, I'm choosing to stay on the optimistic side," said Dr. Abergel.

We were so happy to talk with Dr. Abergel! When we left him, we felt cheered up a little. In the worst of times, God enabled him to inspire hope.

CHAPTER FOURTEEN

Burden Bearers

AFTER ELIZABETH'S TRACHEOTOMY, THE DOCTORS were raring to go into more chest tube therapy. They'd already determined that Elizabeth's biggest trouble spot was her upper left lung. It had quite a significant amount of trapped air and collapse in it. At the top, the lung was 1 ½ inches from the chest wall, and it needed to be much closer. So she was scheduled to have a new, medium-sized chest tube put there that afternoon. The doctors who leaned toward the optimistic side hoped it would help her significantly.

In addition to the phrase "fully re-expanded", we learned more phrases which describe desirable chest tube therapy results—"not fibrotic," "able to expand," and "fully re-inflated." If a lung was able to expand, it meant the air pocket had been removed. That enabled the lung to fill with air properly again. If normal inhaling and exhaling were resumed, it proved extreme scarring was not present.

We received a brief explanation of the steps involved in chest tube therapy. It begins when a tube is inserted into an air pocket within the lung sac to release trapped air and enable it to re-inflate.

Next, suction must be applied in the proper amount to reposition the lung sac and hold it in place. Suction may be increased or decreased to meet specific needs over a period of days or weeks. Applying the proper amount of suction requires a very delicate balance.

Once it's determined that suction is no longer needed, it's turned off. The tube is left in place and that condition is called "water sealed."

When a re-inflated lung sac is water sealed for a good amount of time without the development of any new problems, the chest tube can be removed and the work done by that particular tube is considered successful.

※

Back at home, Maggie was busy creating beautiful prom hairstyles for Sarah and her friend. I could hear the prom dress and ironing board calling my name from home.

It was close to lunch time when Tami returned to sit with Elizabeth. John just happened to arrive at the same time. Matt and I introduced them before we left ICU.

As we drove home, God helped Matt and I adjust into "regular life festivities mode". It was important to Sarah and to us, too. Once I got the dress ironed, Sarah got dressed. She looked stunning! The guys arrived, pictures were taken, and they were off. We were thankful we could be there and at the same time leave Elizabeth in Tami and John's capable hands—no worries.

Matt and I had time to talk alone on the way back to the hospital that evening. It was nice.

"Matt, how do you feel about not mentioning the lung transplant information to Elizabeth all day?" I asked.

"Good," he said. "I think it was the right thing to do. What do you think?"

"I feel the same way," I said. "I think we should we keep it up."

"Yeah, I think that would be good, too," he said.

After talking to Dr. Abergel that morning, we were so thankful we hadn't quickly pounced on Elizabeth with the transplant information. We figured what she didn't know couldn't hurt her. We planned to request that every friend and family member who went in to see her be careful not to mention it as well. What we didn't think of was that it had been written in her file, and nurses and other medical personnel had been reading it.

Tami and John were enjoying time with Elizabeth. However, when her chest tube procedure was about to be done, a nurse sent them back to the waiting room. They waited a good while and then called again to request a visit. After they were denied access to her room, Tami asked John if she could treat him to lunch. Usually, you don't have to ask John that question twice.

The two of them enjoyed getting to know each other immensely during lunch. In no time, their conversation moved into a deeper level, discussing God's purpose for the current trial.

After returning to the ICU waiting room, they tried to get buzzed in to see Elizabeth. Once again, they were denied access. Afternoon began turning to evening, and Tami realized she had to leave. They said "goodbye" and John waited there for our family to return.

After the chest tube procedure was done, an x-ray was taken to check out the results.

"Your lung fully re-expanded!" Elizabeth's excited nurse told her.

When the thoracic surgeon was notified about the fully re-expanded lung, he seemed pleasantly surprised.

"How cool is that?!" he asked.

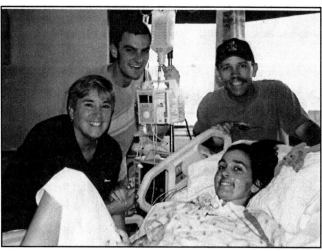

Mom, John, Dad, and Elizabeth loving "cool" news in the Oxnard ICU

As we went through that day, we noticed a quiet, gradual turning away from the authoritative lung transplant pronouncement of the previous night. Instead, the attention of the doctors had been drawn toward chest tube therapy. It had quickly become the new priority, passion, and conversation topic in Elizabeth's case. For the most part, everyone began ignoring the earlier recommendation. Toward the end of the day, it felt like an ominous, threatening cloud was beginning to dissipate instead of worsen.

When big discouragements like the lung transplant recommendation came, negative thoughts forced their way into my mind.

"Maybe God isn't going to heal her," I'd think. "Maybe it's time to give up."

We had no idea what the future would hold. But He didn't let us quit. He never told us He was done working. He never impressed it upon us to stop praying. He just picked us up, provided new encouragement and strength, and helped us face the new problems.

At one point that night, I was sitting by myself in the waiting room. There were many other families talking with each other in the room. I had my Bible with me, and I began reading in the book of Psalms. I found a verse that grabbed my attention.

> "Once God has spoken, twice I have heard this: that power belongs to God (Psalm 62:11 NASB).

I blocked out the noise around me and just sat there thinking about power belonging to God—*all* power—power to do anything! Then my mind shifted to lung transplant thoughts. After a little while, the Holy Spirit spoke a sentence silently, yet authoritatively into my mind and spirit.

You're not going to need that.

That sentence was so clearly and powerfully impressed on my mind. I knew God just told me His plan on the lung transplant issue. I treasured those six words and pondered them. It was so special; I didn't tell anyone else about it for a long time.

When they had prepared to insert the new chest tube that afternoon, they promised Elizabeth they'd manage her pain effectively. They gave her good amounts of pain medication, but afterward, she wrote a note telling us that the medicine didn't effectively numb the pain. She went through the procedure without much help. She was awake when they inserted the chest tube into her lung and she heard it make a high pitched sound.

Shortly after she was returned to her ICU room, the chest tube was attached to a source of suction. The suction generated more intense pain which lasted for a couple of days or so.

As her lungs re-inflated or fully re-expanded, Elizabeth began to experience an additional source of extreme pain. We were told that there were many sensitive nerve ends called alveoli inside the lung sacs. As the lung sacs began to move back into their proper positions after being even partly collapsed for weeks, it could be extremely painful. And it was.

The new medical staff tried to help her with pain medication, but they didn't seem to know she'd already had tons of drugs and had developed a tolerance for them before being transferred. That brought frustration.

The doctors cared about Elizabeth's pain, but more than that, they wanted her lungs to improve. One doctor reminded her again—it was just going to hurt, but that it wouldn't hurt anymore once she was well.

The following afternoon, many of Elizabeth's friends from Biola came to visit. They hadn't seen her in over a month. The "lung transplant report" really hit them all hard, too. It was the weekend before their finals and they made a huge sacrifice of study time to come. So many friends came, we had to find another waiting room. We scouted around and found one not in use on the first floor.

Friends rotated in and out of her room, packing her afternoon with joy, encouragement, and laughter. She was so happy to see each of them, and every friend was thrilled to have time with her. Some couldn't hold back tears of joy, thankfulness, and amazement. When we visited her later, Elizabeth was tired, yet overjoyed. She'd been so blessed. That day, she'd seen God bring two verses from Psalms to life dramatically in her hospital room.

> "I said to the Lord, 'You are my Lord; apart from you I have no good thing.' As for the saints who are in the land,

they are the glorious ones in whom is all my delight" (Psalm 16:2–3).

The two-to three-week time recommendation to do chest tube therapy gave us more time to pray for God to continue the healing He'd begun over a month ago. Dr. Abergel shared an update with us after Elizabeth's first few days in Oxnard.

"She's improving…she looks good," he said. "I'm pleased with the way things are looking. The early chest tube efforts are going well. I'm optimistic she won't need lung transplantation."

Then he shared his thoughts about it.

"Lung transplantation is a big ordeal," he said.

The phrase "big ordeal" when we were already in one didn't sound too appealing to me.

"It's not some perfect, quick-fix for problems like the ones Elizabeth faces," he added. "I really feel the course of treatment we're using will have a better long-range outcome."

God continued showing us that every new danger or fear had to be faced with faith and prayer. Each answer we received along the way was significant. After three days of prayer about lung transplantation, we saw another astonishing answer from God. The thoracic surgeon started to move away from his earlier position. God dealt with the most recent threat for Elizabeth in a better, more amazing way. In answer to our prayers, God was changing those lungs and helping one doctor gain a new, hopeful perspective. Incredible!

Since moving to the Oxnard hospital, Elizabeth had been busy with procedures. When we saw things slow down a bit, we figured it was a good time to decorate her room. Her nurse said we could put up whatever we wanted. So we taped many cheery cards and pictures on her walls and windows where she could see them best. Elizabeth gave directions on placement preferences. By that time, her pile of get well cards was quite large and it kept increasing. Two of her prayer supporters were school teachers who sent loads of sweet pictures and cards made by their kindergarten and middle school students.

We also taped up photographs of family members, friends, and other well-wishers among the cards. One of my personal favorites was a set of enlargements of pictures Jeri took back on April 23rd, the night Elizabeth's chance of survival percentage first moved from 50% to 70%. In the pictures, we all had huge smiles, extreme joy, and a few made enthusiastic "thumbs-up" gestures. Elizabeth still didn't know the exact significance of the joy in the pictures, but they were very uplifting. Each item put on her wall was special, and we had fun arranging an awesome display.

Since her transfer there, Elizabeth faced the new, sharp, ongoing pain of additional chest tubes without pain medication potency, and the illusive goal of extubation. We definitely sensed an increased need for prayer. We knew many people were praying all the time. But gathering in a concentrated, united time was powerful in a unique way. We scheduled another nighttime prayer session two days later. The hospital had a beautiful chapel we could use. We got the word out: "Elizabeth needs more prayer. Please come pray with us."

I knew the Biola University semester would end soon and graduation would take place in a couple of days. It would have been Elizabeth's graduation. I sent a thank you e-mail to the university, since they'd given her so much support.

"Dearest Biola University: The entire family of Elizabeth McGovern is full of gratitude for your tireless, passionate work of prayer during her illness. Through your prayers, God has already brought her through many dangers, toils, and snares. We stand in awe of Him with you. Through all of this, God is teaching us that power belongs to Him and that He alone is due all the glory for all He has done.

"He has assembled her doctors, nurses, and respiratory therapists and He has used them mightily in many ways. Each improvement in her condition, whether large or small, brings such joy. And each setback brings the new realization that this time of illness and waiting is designed by

Him for His own good reasons and it is fully in His hands, timing, and authority. We can rest in Him.

"Thank you, again, for your prayer support and love for Elizabeth in Christ. May each of you have a summer full of the joy of His presence and the satisfaction of fulfilling the purposes of His great and wise heart in your own life. Praying with you for Elizabeth's full recovery, in the deep, deep love of Jesus,

Matt, Diane, Maggie and Sarah McGovern"

The next morning was the beginning of Elizabeth's 42nd day in the hospital. The medical staff discussed Elizabeth's case during their rounds. Apparently, the improvements and change of direction into aggressive chest tube therapy over the past week had not been written in her chart. The recommendation for a lung transplant was the most recent entry. And since the entire medical staff was rarely present at the same time during rounds, people who worked in ICU weren't always on the same page.

So, not long after rounds, Elizabeth's nurse for the day came into her room.

"It's a good day for your transfer to UCLA," he said cheerfully.

Sadly, a doctor who'd been only marginally involved in her care since April, had written an order to transfer her to UCLA that day for a lung transplant.

Elizabeth seemed surprised, and I felt panicky.

"Can I talk to you outside?" I asked the nurse.

We walked to an area out of earshot of Elizabeth's room.

"There isn't going to be a transfer today to UCLA or anywhere else," I said. "Her doctor has begun chest tube therapy instead of pursuing a transplant."

"But the transfer for a lung transplant order is definitely in her file," he said confidently. He insisted that a decision had been made.

"I wonder if he knows something I don't," I thought. "Matt and I haven't heard a word about a transfer all week. I don't believe a decision like this can be made entirely without us."

The nurse seemed so sure of his information. He didn't back down at all. The nurse and I were caught in an oppressive confusion.

None of the doctors who'd been involved in her recent chest tube work were present at morning rounds. I felt frustrated, angry, and helpless. The muddled communication was highly unacceptable to me. But at that moment, we didn't see how the conflict could be resolved. I wanted Dr. Abergel.

Until this was cleared up, my solution was to tell the nurse that my husband and I had decided not to mention the lung transplant idea to Elizabeth unless it became necessary.

"I don't want you to mention it to her again," I said firmly.

When I returned to Elizabeth's room, I realized I was stuck. I had to give her an explanation. She knew something was up since I'd asked the nurse to leave the room to talk to me.

"He doesn't know what he's talking about," I said. "When the doctors were discussing your case a week ago, one doctor suggested you get a lung transplant. But then, within one or two days, they changed their position on it and started the chest tube work instead."

I started to think seriously that the time may have come to tell her the whole truth. It was getting too hard keeping up our "encouragement only" communication system. She desperately wanted answers.

That unsettling conflict crushed my spirit. The situation seemed so unnecessary to me. I'd been in her room almost every day, was quite aware of her treatment, and I was her mother.

"Why won't the nurse believe me?" I asked myself. "I really feel this young nurse doesn't have his facts straight! How can this be fixed?"

I had to get away and think. I took a long walk outside around the entire hospital, but no solution came to me. I felt drained.

I was still very bothered as I walked back inside, so I almost leapt for joy when I saw Dr. Abergel standing in the hall outside of ICU. I told him about the conflict, and he reassured me they couldn't transfer Elizabeth without talking to us first.

Within a half hour, the ICU nurse supervisor came to talk with me in the waiting room. I assumed Dr. Abergel had spoken to her. She was caring, compassionate, and calm when I wasn't. She asked questions and listened well.

"Conflicts abound in a hospital this size, and quite often doctors hold varied opinions on treatment or procedures," she explained. "If the doctors are confused or conflicted, it trickles down to the nurses. We try to get everyone on the same page during rounds, but problems like yours still happen."

After the conflict with the nurse, I felt wrung out emotionally. I was absolutely ready to drop. But that evening we'd scheduled the prayer gathering for our friends and family. I was not up to spending time with the treasured company making its way to the hospital chapel. Honestly, I didn't feel much like praying. I felt like I couldn't carry my burden anymore, but I was sure these friends weren't as tired as I was. I counted on their spiritual fervency. I needed them to bear my burden for a bit so I could stand up again.

God assembled precious believers that night.

"You care and you're here!" I thought as I greeted each one and watched them take a seat.

We knew they'd taken time out of their busy schedules to be with us. Matt and I felt so blessed and comforted by each faithful soul who came to pray.

There was a peculiar beauty to long-range perseverance in prayer for a massive need. We saw it on the faces of these friends. Among other things, it called for sheer-dogged determination. They'd already been praying for one and a half months with us. Their presence spoke volumes!

The focus of our prayer time was two-fold. First and foremost—Elizabeth's body truly needed more almighty power to heal it. We knew our God was the One to ask. We'd pray big. But secondly, her family and John required endurance. We wanted to be upheld, sustained, and reinforced to continue on in our journey with her. These believers stood by us that night and kept us from drowning in our dilemma.

Before we prayed together, I read a couple of verses from a psalm that fit our situation perfectly that day.

> "The righteous cry out, and the Lord hears them; He delivers them from all their troubles. The Lord is close to the brokenhearted and saves those who are crushed in spirit. A righteous man may have many troubles, but the Lord delivers him from them all" (Psalm 34:17–19).

As we prepared to pray, Elizabeth was lying in her bed one floor above us. We began lifting her specific needs up to God yet again. By faith, we petitioned the Lord for His healing hand to touch her body and ease her agonizing pain. We requested His help for every specific need He brought to our hearts and minds.

As we moved through that season of prayer, the Holy Spirit transfused us with faith and hope again. God used His people to throw us a life preserver. Righteous men and women uniting in prayer was clearly powerful and effective.

When we visited Elizabeth after our prayer session, she was still in great pain from the chest tube therapy and there wasn't a whole lot they could do about it. But she persevered. God made her strong in her spirit so she could endure it.

As we drove home that night, my mind went back to a time two years earlier, another time of "leaving." That time we were leaving Elizabeth at Biola as a new student. It was the first time she'd be living away from home.

I felt nervous to say my final goodbye. Parents of college students tend to get like that! Our family walked together to the street outside her dorm. The time had come. Before leaving, Elizabeth and I sadly gave each other a long hug.

"I love you so much," I said as tears filled my eyes.

"I love you, too, Mom," she proclaimed with tears running down her cheeks.

I almost burst out with loud sobs, but somehow I held them back. It was hard to walk away from her at Biola back then. I realized, now, that leaving her in such awful pain in a hospital bed was much harder.

The next morning, a new respiratory therapist came in to check Elizabeth's ventilator settings and saw that she was having a hard time. Her beautiful, compassionate heart was moved to comfort Elizabeth. She spoke tenderly and even cried with her.

Many times, when people met Elizabeth, they liked her immediately and longed to do everything possible to help her get better. The Lord prompted them to share strong hope and encouragement with her. He still directed total strangers to pray for her.

Friends and family kept sending cards with encouraging comments and scripture verses. Nancy and her husband, Frank, sent a card with a Bible verse inside.

"I will be glad and rejoice in your love, for you saw my affliction and knew the anguish of my soul" (Psalm 31:7).

Another relative reported the prayer support her church was giving Elizabeth.

"We haven't stopped naming Elizabeth's name before the throne of the Heavenly Father since we heard of her illness," she said. "The name 'Elizabeth' has spread far and wide midst the Body of Christ."

The power of the praying Body of Christ carried her along.

Since the transfer, Elizabeth had missed the nice TV and VCR arrangement she'd had back at Camarillo. In a facility that size, that kind of setup was hard to find outside the children's ward. But, amazingly, a kind chaplain was able to arrange it for her.

That night, Elizabeth and John created what became known as a "bedside movie date." Our family went home early so they could be alone. Just before their "date" began, John slid a chair as close to Elizabeth as he could. After putting in the video they'd chosen to watch, he sat down at the side of her bed.

The nurses allowed John to stay a little past the end of visiting hours so they could finish watching their movie. It seemed everyone was supportive of their developing romance.

When we returned home that night, we listened to an answering machine message in response to my recent e-mail. It was from Clyde Cook.

"I just want to thank you so much for sending me a copy of the letter to the Biola family regarding Elizabeth," he said. "I've been praying for her and this was an encouraging letter to me, because I'd heard that she was really struggling there for a while in it. So just let her know that I am praying and that the whole Biola family knows about it and is praying.

"We're getting ready for commencement in just about an hour and a half and the graduation then tomorrow. It's kind of an exciting time here at Biola, and yet our hearts are with Elizabeth."

He closed his message with a prayer.

"Father, I just lift up Elizabeth before you, again. Just touch her and bring healing. Father, those lungs belong to you and I just pray that you'd do all that you need to do—your special divine touch to bring her back to full strength and health. I pray for all the family and friends she has at Biola as they stand alongside and lift her up to the throne of grace where there's help and mercy in time of need. So we commit her and the family to you. Amen."

CHAPTER FIFTEEN

The Shepherd's Voice

A FEW DAYS LATER, RELATIVES from both sides of our family came to visit Elizabeth. She'd come a long way since their previous visits and each pair that entered her room was excited to see her awake, smiling and writing notes. They were thrilled to see the change made by the tracheotomy. Even in pain, she looked so much better to them. Each relative returned to the waiting room full of joy and excitement. Their enthusiasm rekindled our own.

The believers prayed on. Many of the daily prayer requests that we'd begun e-mailing were repeated because progress slowed down or stopped quite often. I looked for new ways to word them. Two special phrases described the desire of our hearts for Elizabeth's recovery that week: "significant improvements" and "substantial improvements." We forged ahead and asked God for big progress.

John felt it was time to get back to Biola to take his finals. That night, he and Elizabeth shared a meaningful time of note-writing/talking before he left.

"Before I got sick, I asked the Lord to make me more patient," she wrote. "Through all of this, God has really been teaching me about patience and perseverance. This isn't what I expected, but God is working. He's funny. Now I don't want to be patient any more."

The last note was a short dialogue between the two of them.
John: "You are an awesome woman…"
Elizabeth: "Thank you. You are awesome, too."

In their final moments together that night, Elizabeth hated even thinking about John leaving. Saying goodbye again was painful.

When John returned to the waiting room, he was quite excited.

"What a woman! What a woman!" he kept exclaiming joyfully.

Elizabeth's faith and beauty were easy to see. He seemed even more fascinated with her that night than he'd been before.

The next week, Dr. Abergel rotated back in to care for Elizabeth. Just having him there always made us feel better. However, he was aggressive when he felt it was needed, which made things tougher on Elizabeth.

"It's time to increase normal physical movement because it will help push her lungs further into recovery," he said. "I'll tell the physical therapists to step it up."

The first physical challenge was to get Elizabeth into a sitting position again. She'd been lying in a bed for one month and twelve days, so sitting up would be a huge accomplishment. It required all the lung functioning she could muster, even briefly. None of us was there when her first attempt was made. The physical therapists held her up by the shoulders for ten minutes that day. Whether she felt like it or not, she had to get moving. "Rise up, oh woman of God!"

John and I were first up to visit Elizabeth the next morning. As we entered the ICU, we could see her room in the distance and we saw a dark-haired person sitting in a chair to the side of her bed. It surprised us. We walked all the way across ICU to her room.

"Who is that person?" we both wondered.

We walked in and saw it was Elizabeth and our mouths dropped open. All we could do was stare! We were blown away! Her bed was empty and she was sitting in a chair. It took a little while to process the event. I continued staring at that empty bed.

John and I knew "substantial" when we saw it! We'd prayed for big improvements, and were delighted to suddenly see one. The two of us eventually closed our mouths, sat on the bed, and visited with her. We couldn't wait to tell everyone else!

It wasn't long before Maggie and I got to watch Elizabeth perform her second physical challenge. We happened to be in her room the following morning when her physical therapists showed up. They said we could stay if we moved to the side of her room. Then they prepared Elizabeth for action. While carefully maneuvering around her chest tubes and monitor boxes, they unhooked her from the ventilator and hooked her up to a portable oxygen supply for a workout.

Suddenly Maggie and I saw it! Our tall, elegant Elizabeth was raised up to a sitting position with help, her legs were moved to the side of the bed, and she prepared to stand. They placed a walker in front of her for stability. She was helped to her feet and then she slowly began taking incredible steps—five steps forward/five steps backward—two times. That day, she took a total of 20 steps.

Our hearts pounded with excitement and huge, amazed smiles covered our faces! Maggie and I looked at Elizabeth with great joy and pride. Seeing that significant piece of her recovery history in the making was so encouraging!

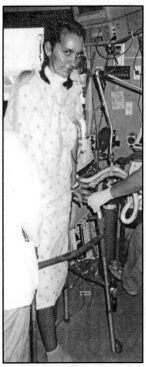

One of Elizabeth's first steps

After twelve days of chest tube therapy, Elizabeth had a total of five chest tubes in her lungs. Two of them were the original ones that had been inserted way back on Day 1. Five chest tubes plus a new hand-held suction tube created a patient who continually required great amounts of suction. She used the suction tube so much, it was like a permanent addition to her hand. Our ears had grown accustomed to the frequent sound of it in her room. We knew if you loved someone, you had to accept them as they were—warts, suction, and all. After all, "love means never having to say you're sorry for having suction needs."

Matt stayed diligent with his chest tube inspection work in the Oxnard hospital. As a scientist, he went after answers quickly if he saw any change. He'd report it to a nurse or a doctor and keep asking about it until he got an explanation. However, with Matt's work schedule, there were more hours of the day when he wasn't there to do his inspections. And it had become more challenging, since Elizabeth had more chest tubes and monitor boxes than before.

One morning when Matt was gone, Elizabeth and I saw John pick up the tube inspection task all on his own. No one asked him to do it; he just knew. I guess it was a guy thing. Much like Matt, John circled the entire bed and carefully examined each tube and monitor box. Matt and John, the chest tube men, were important.

With these tubes in place and receiving suction, Elizabeth's lungs experienced both progress and pain. At best, medication only took the edge off the pain. Varying levels of extreme pain were her constant companion. Elizabeth bore it well, not with complaints, tears, or angry, helpless outbursts. She persevered bravely. She was amazing, my hero.

Shortly after we arrived in Elizabeth's room the next morning, the thoracic surgeon came in. He looked over a few things.

"Her lungs are fully up," he reported happily. "They re-inflated."

"Excellent!" I said.

"It's better than excellent!" he countered.

Then he announced what he was about to do—turn off the suction on four of the five tubes, the condition called "water sealed." He also said he hoped to start removing some tubes a few days later. When I heard his plan, I made a silly outburst.

"Happy, happy, happy, happy, boing, boing, boing, boing!" I said.

It was a joyful celebration phrase from "Sesame Street" that flashed across my mind.

"Did I just say that in front of a brilliant heart surgeon?" I quickly asked myself.

After he turned off suction to the four tubes, it went fine.

Later that morning, doctors began making their own joyful celebration phrases of a more grown-up nature.

"She's looking great!"

"Her x-ray looks fabulous!"

"This is the best I've seen her yet!"

"Her lungs are fully re-expanded!" (always a favorite).

"She's so much improved!"

The medical staff seemed very enthusiastic about her progress. I couldn't believe what I was hearing.

"Am I dreaming?" I asked myself.

However, as I watched the chest tube process, I began to sense that chest tube work was not an exact science. It included a lot of trial and error. Miscalculations or mistakes could be made.

I also started grasping the fact that if a lung was fully re-inflated at one time, it might not stay that way indefinitely. Things changed frequently. One air pocket could clear up, but a new one would develop nearby. Nevertheless, overall improvement took place.

One example of the unpredictable nature of chest tube therapy was demonstrated at the end of the third week. A new problem developed—the larger chest tube in her right lung became loose and fell out. Consequently, Dr. Abergel began watching the right lung, since it looked like a new air pocket was already developing there.

The next day, the pneumothorax in the right lung was worse. It had become a little larger and some collapse had occurred. Dr. Abergel felt she'd need a new chest tube in her right lung. They also saw another problem in the left lung which meant she might require an additional chest tube there, too.

Later that afternoon, Maggie and I were in Elizabeth's room again. The two of them visited on one side of her bed while I sat alone on the other. Suddenly, a doctor I hadn't met before entered her room. The girls didn't notice him or hear what he said. He spoke directly to me and reported a new finding.

His news wasn't good. He was sure his report meant big trouble for Elizabeth's lungs.

"She'll never make progress or be able to get off the ventilator because her lungs are too destroyed," he insisted. "The chest tube therapy will never work." He stubbornly maintained his hopeless outlook—whatever Elizabeth's body needed to do, it wasn't able to do. His words sounded so final. He made me feel like the only intelligent thing to do would be to give up.

Then he left as abruptly as he'd entered.

I'd heard many things like that before. I was aware my dependence on God had been weakening some since her transfer to Oxnard. After he left, I allowed myself to really think long and hard about his words.

That's where I went wrong. I tried to listen to a voice I didn't know. John 10:2–5 does a perfect job of explaining voice recognition that leads to following Jesus.

> "The man who enters by the gate is the shepherd of his sheep. The watchman opens the gate for him, and the sheep listen to his voice. He calls his own sheep by name and leads them out. When he has brought out all his own, he goes on ahead of them, and the sheep follow him because they know his voice. But they will never follow a stranger; in fact they will run away from him because they do not recognize a stranger's voice."

Instead of realizing I'd heard a "stranger's voice," I allowed this man's words and adamant tone to run through my mind repeatedly. As a consequence, a heaviness started pressing down on my spirit. Despair was near.

In the middle of that struggle, God spoke to my spirit.

Don't you remember I've been teaching you not to believe these people right off when they tell you things like this? He asked me. *I don't want you to think like that doctor.*

He led me to confess that I was forgetting all He'd been doing so far. I felt bad. It amazed me to realize how easily I could forget the recent actions of my awesome God.

After that, He quietly reminded me He was in charge and pointed out my greatest need.

You must get your thoughts back on Me, listen to My voice, and trust Me alone.

When I heard His voice again, I joyfully recognized it. Then God recharged my memory so I could think straight. Truths flowed through my mind once again.

"I'm only safe with my mind on God," I thought. "I must reject this strange voice and take these thoughts captive...His voice is the only one that makes sense...If God wants to, He will enable Elizabeth to, again, do what seems humanly impossible."

While I sat quietly in my chair, His peace returned. I felt the Lord lift my burden off of me! My heart and mind were free. I recalled the many times He'd tried to teach me the same lesson since April. But with me, much repetition was still required. I remembered how it had been all the way through. God only sent thoughts with hope. The utter despair never came from Him.

The unpredictability of chest tube therapy persisted. By the following morning, the two dark areas they'd seen on her x-ray the day before had vanished. Dr. Abergel told Elizabeth the good news that she wouldn't need another tube, after all. So she and the medical staff were really "up" that day.

About mid-morning, things had slowed down a bit in her room. Everything grew quiet, and I looked around and saw that both Elizabeth and Maggie had fallen asleep. A fan rotated my way and sent a brief, cool push of wind.

My attention was drawn to the good, beautiful, strong numbers I saw on Elizabeth's monitor. I was full of gratitude.

As I stared joyfully at her monitor, I recalled the serious jeopardy each number had been in for so many weeks. I knew those numbers had been passionately prayed for, longed for, ached for. Every single one of them indicated improved breathing and the healing power of a mighty God.

I had a clear view of Elizabeth's chest as it rose and fell while she breathed comfortably. What a beautiful sight! My mind jumped back again to the beginning of her illness—to her painful, stooped over breathing the night we entered the ER. What a comparison! I was overwhelmed! Then the Spirit stirred me to a prayer of praise.

"Lord, you've done so much in Elizabeth's broken, young body," I prayed. "I am amazed, relieved, hopeful, fearful. You alone work wonders! Thank you *so much* Father."

After Elizabeth woke up from her brief nap, she looked out at the view from her room.

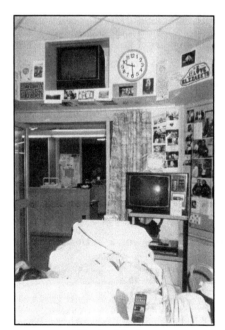

Elizabeth's view

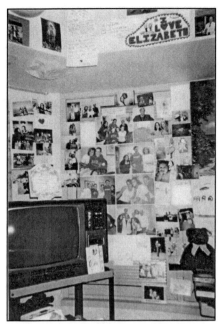

Some ICU room wall art

Occasionally, someone would encourage Elizabeth to write in a journal, but inspiration for that rarely came. Instead, she liked writing brief notes and we loved every word. That morning, she suddenly felt the desire to write "thank you" notes and decorate them with hand-drawn hearts for her family members. Since green is Elizabeth's favorite color, she always chose to write her notes with a green marker. Then she personally delivered her special, individual cards to us. Matt and I quickly cherished the one we shared.

"I just want to thank you for all your prayers and support. You have been so patient and encouraging through this hard time. I really appreciate it. I don't think I could have survived this far without God and you. Thank you for all your dedication. You are the best Mom and Dad. You have been such a good witness, too. I love you both so much. Thanks again. Elizabeth"

That day the chaplain came by for a brief visit. He told Elizabeth she'd done what he'd been unable to do for years. He mentioned that one of the doctors working on her case had never had an open mind about God.

"You've made a change in that a little," he told her.

Elizabeth just smiled at him and pointed upward.

Late the following afternoon, one extremely helpful respiratory therapist arrived with a Passy-Muir Valve (PMV—our abbreviation) that had been ordered the week before. It was a small, plastic device about the size of a dime that they would attach to Elizabeth's trach tube to work on strengthening an area of her lungs.

When the respiratory therapist ordered it, she'd told us of a possible and delightful side effect—it could conceivably enable her to talk again while on the ventilator. Since we heard that, we'd been selfishly longing to hear her voice.

Weeks ago, we'd been told Elizabeth could have permanent vocal chord damage since she'd remained on the ventilator for an extended period. We were hoping and praying that after all these weeks, those vocal chords would still work.

Matt, John, and Sarah were actually the ones in Elizabeth's room when the respiratory therapist attached the little plastic cap to the end of her trach tube for the first time. All eyes and ears in the room were on Elizabeth. As they looked on expectantly, she spoke her first words in close to two months.

"Hi. Thank you all for helping me."

Knowing Maggie and I would want to be a part of the excitement, John and Sarah decided to fetch us from the waiting room. As they were leaving her room to get us, Elizabeth called out to them.

"I love you guys!"

"Wow! Elizabeth is talking again!" they thought.

Then John and Sarah raced into the waiting room all wild-eyed and told us what had just happened. Maggie and I got in there as fast as we could. We stared and listened intently as Elizabeth talked.

Her words started out soft and a little raspy, but her voice had tone to it. We loved hearing anything she had to say. The respiratory therapist was all smiles. Any medical personnel that came by listened in and smiled, too.

Maggie and I stayed in her room longer than we realized. We totally forgot about Sarah and John who wanted to get back in as soon as possible. We just kept staring with amazement.

I read the booklet that accompanied the valve, and I was impressed by its inventor—a ventilator-dependent man, David A. Muir. He desired the highest quality of life involvement for people in his same situation.

I was moved by the goal of the company that produced it, which was summarized by Patricia E. Passy.

> "We at Passy-Muir, Inc. believe that communication is the essence of the human spirit; it is essential to individual rights and dignity. We are committed in our efforts to offer tracheostomized and ventilator-dependent patients a step toward independence and dignity through speech."[11]

Elizabeth noticed that the Passy-Muir Valve made her lungs work a little harder. She usually didn't welcome changes like that, even if they would help her, but her respiratory therapists persevered. They attached the valve periodically and then removed it later, much like other ventilator adjustments.

While she had the valve attached that first evening, we made a phone call to one of her grandmas to let her hear Elizabeth's voice. It was strangely wonderful seeing Elizabeth talk on a phone again. Her grandmother was delighted to receive her brief call.

We were so thankful for the help of the respiratory therapist and a little plastic cap from a wonderful man named David A. Muir.

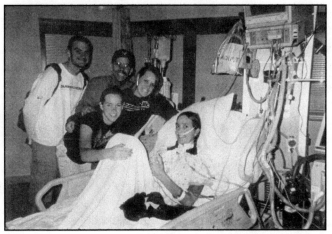

John, Sarah, Matt, and Maggie happy to hear Elizabeth's voice again

---

11   Passage courtesy of Passy-Muir, Inc., Irvine, CA.

When I arrived the next morning with Maggie and John, I felt fresh, rested, and optimistic. As I entered ICU, I saw Dr. Abergel on my way to Elizabeth's room.

"I have new concerns for her right lung," he said. "It has collapsed some again, so we *do* need to put in another chest tube. I already talked to Elizabeth."

"She's had setbacks before," I said in response to that unwanted news. "This is just another one."

I signed the procedure authorization for insertion of another chest tube without giving it much thought. It was scheduled for the afternoon.

But when Elizabeth had heard the news, she knew another chest tube meant much more pain and time required on suction. She appeared crushed the moment we entered her room. It was heartbreaking to see her so down.

The three of us spent some unhurried time rotating around reading portions of the Word to her that God laid on our hearts. She carefully listened, as usual. Then we prayed for her around her bed. We stuck by her during her "waiting for more pain" morning.

Whenever Elizabeth experienced new discouragement, we gave all we had to encourage her, which left us drained again. It was a continual cycle. We eventually left for lunch, but on the way back, the Lord used one of our favorite Shane and Shane worship songs to strengthen us again. We sang along with it in the car. Its phrases lifted our spirits.

"Praise the name of Jesus, praise the name of Jesus.

He's my rock, He's my fortress, He's my deliverer

In Him will I trust. Praise the name of Jesus."[12]

I took the CD into Elizabeth's room and played it for her when we got back. She knew and loved the song, too. While we sang it together, it helped refocus us on Jesus.

About mid-afternoon, we learned the doctors had discovered another air pocket in her left lung. So Elizabeth's early morning report of "needing one more chest tube" turned into "needing two more chest tubes."

---

12 "Praise the Name of Jesus," words and music by Roy Hicks, Jr., © 1976, Latter Rain Music (ASCAP) (adm. at EMICMGPublishing.com). All rights reserved. Used by permission.

As Elizabeth faced more tubes and more pain, she had to stand up against *her* greatest enemy on her journey—discouragement. The peace of God ruled in her heart, but it took brutal hits from discouragement. Because she'd been in a coma during the first crucial days of her illness, she'd bypassed the fear of her death. But what she feared now was never getting better, never getting off the ventilator, never going home.

The procedure was done around 3:30. As usual, the promised pain medication didn't work. It was a nightmare for her to be awake, feeling the chest tubes painfully poked into her lungs.

After the procedure, her pain began to intensify. Seeing Elizabeth in such awful pain again and knowing we couldn't do anything to help her swamped us once more.

"Lord, this is too much!" I thought.

Later that afternoon we had a few minutes alone with Dr. Abergel, and he shared what was on his heart.

"Caring for a chronically ill patient like Elizabeth is frustrating, draining, and absolutely exhausting!" he said.

The doctors wanted her well very badly. They were trying everything they could. That was the only time I sensed discouragement in him.

"But I can't wait for 'her day' to come," he added. "When 'her day' comes, she'll get off the ventilator for good and out of the hospital.

He longed for "her day" as much as we did.

CHAPTER SIXTEEN

Longsuffering

SARAH AND I VISITED WITH Elizabeth the next morning. After a while, the respiratory therapist attached the PMV. For many weeks, Elizabeth had grown quite aware that information was sometimes kept from her. Remaining uninformed was torturing her.

"What happened to me?" she asked all of a sudden.

"Do you really want to know?" I asked.

"Yes," she said.

I decided to go ahead. I started by telling her she'd had such a bad case of viral pneumonia she almost died a couple of times. It was hard putting that into words. Then Sarah and I gave her all the complete answers to previously glossed-over information. We told her great stories of countless answers to prayer. We reported how awesome God had been. We filled in all the details about the thoracic surgeon's lung transplant recommendation and the conflict I had with the nurse about it over a month earlier.

"Never getting any information was so frustrating!" Elizabeth said.

"It was hard to keep things from you, but the doctors and nurses insisted on it—first, because you were such a critical patient and, second—because you'd faced loads of discouragement and pain along your journey," I explained.

"It was wise keeping some of the frightening truth from me," she said. "Thank you for doing that."

The three of us had a great talk. It felt so good to have the restraints lifted.

"Ahhhhh!" I said with a huge exhale. "What a relief!"

<hr />

Ongoing chest tube progress enabled slow, steady improvements toward the goal of getting her off the ventilator. She'd gradually adjusted to a lower setting on the ventilator and eventually, Dr. Abergel felt she was ready for the next and final step—time off the ventilator.

She sustained her first attempt for ten minutes comfortably. Her second trouble-free attempt the following day lasted thirty-five minutes. So far, so good.

Of course, constant, intense pain accompanied her progress. It signified her lung muscles were receiving a workout and being strengthened. As she endured her pain, she remained patient and strong. We saw pain on her face, days without end. We watched her ask for pain medication many, many times.

Occasionally, ventilator work came to a screeching halt if Elizabeth developed a new fever or hospital-acquired infection. She told us once that whenever she got sick again, it made her feel ten times worse and drained all energy from her. Sometimes they had to temporarily move her back to less-challenging ventilator settings. Pseudomonas was the infection she battled most often. By that time, all we had to do was look at her and we could spot a fever coming on.

<hr />

The next morning, Maggie and Sarah's work schedules synchronized briefly so the three of us visited Elizabeth together. Overnight her pain had gone deeper than I thought it could go. It was so hard to see her that way. I began to experience periods of despondency. It felt like we were sinking into a quagmire where we'd have to watch her in pain endlessly.

Before the girls had to leave for work, we got a quick lunch. Just after we finished eating, the Lord gave us a new, unexpected coping mechanism called "silliness."

It all happened after we cleared our trash away. I got out a penny from my purse and put it on the table in front of me. I held it upright on its edge with my thumbs and forefingers. Then, I snapped it forward quickly with my right thumb and forefinger while my left thumb and forefinger provided some resistance in the opposite direction. The penny left my hands and spun fast over the tabletop and we enjoyed it immensely. Eventually, it lost momentum and stopped spinning. I spun it again and again. It made Maggie and Sarah happy. We smiled. We laughed. They asked for pennies of their own.

Once all three of us got our pennies spinning, the fun increased. We were laughing and making loud, excited comments. Occasionally one of our pennies went off the table edge and we'd go after it. We laughed about that, too.

Sadly, we weren't too aware of other people around us. We were so immersed in Elizabeth's pain. I'm sure we were too loud and probably looked ridiculous. But it was a release and we needed it. We noticed it again. Humor temporarily helped relieve the emotional agony of our situation. Just remembering that time makes the three of us smile and laugh.

Consistently walking in faith became harder for me as the time wore on. I'd recently resumed cooking dinner at home for my family. As I drove home that afternoon, I realized I needed encouragement again. So I played a CD by Avalon entitled "The Creed." One song began to play that I'd never heard before—"You Were There." Many of the words fit our experience perfectly.

"I wonder how it must have felt when David stood to face Goliath on a hill. I imagine that he shook with all his might until You took his hand, and held on tight."

At various places within the song, the chorus reminded me that God was always there through it all.

"You were there, you were there in the midst of danger's snare," "when the hardest fight seemed so out of reach," "in the midst of the unclear," "when obedience seemed to not make sense."

And the song ended with words that portray awesome mental pictures of our God.

> "You were the Victor and the King. You were the power in David's swing. You were the calm in Abraham. You were

the God who understands. You are our strength when we have none. You are the living, Holy one."[13]

The song gave me such a clear reminder of the miracles God had already done. I'd experienced His presence all along the way. He *was* always there. Fresh thoughts of God's power and omnipresence filled me up with new hope and joy. I listened to the song repeatedly so I could learn the beautiful words. Then I sang along with the CD with all my heart.

Having a loved one in ICU had the uncanny ability to take us quite high one moment, and then way down in the pits the next. We couldn't get off the lung disease recovery roller coaster with Elizabeth. Her ups and downs continued to affect us deeply. I'd just been richly blessed by the song, but a sudden, extreme drop happened again within a few hours.

After my family had shared a nice meal at home, we drove back for the evening visit. For some reason, we all (except John) quickly got on each others' nerves quite a bit. Each of us said mean things and provoked one another.

By the time we parked the car, we were done talking. We were all so mad—again, with the exception of John—that we didn't even want to walk next to each other on the way into the hospital. The car doors opened and we all scattered—frustrated and annoyed. Each of us walked in alone. It took two to three minutes to get from the parking lot to the ICU and we needed a few minutes to calm down. We then gathered together in the ICU waiting room. Even at our worst, we knew we needed to stick by Elizabeth. We knew she needed us and we needed her.

John wisely said nothing as he saw our family temporarily fall apart and turn on each other. He'd learned it was all a part of the journey God had sent us on together.

---

[13] "You Were There," words by Benjamin Glover, © 2004, Extended Stay Music, (ASCAP) (admin. by The Loving Company). All Rights Reserved. Used By Permission.

I needed some time alone the next morning, so Maggie went to visit Elizabeth while I slept in a little. Then I set out to run a few errands and breathe in non-hospital air for an hour or two.

I was totally enjoying myself at the mall when Maggie called and said Elizabeth was in immense pain again. She needed to leave for work soon and didn't want to leave Elizabeth alone that way. So I dropped the remainder of my plans and quickly drove back to the hospital.

When I arrived, Elizabeth was in tons of dreadful pain. I tried to figure out the cause. The day before, she stayed off the ventilator for four hours, which was a long stretch of time for her. I wondered if it had been too much of a lung workout in one day.

Sarah's high school graduation was the following day. John planned to skip it and stay with Elizabeth that day so we'd all feel okay about not visiting. He was so good about finding ways to help. A couple of days earlier, Tami heard us discussing graduation plans and she volunteered to stay with Elizabeth that day, too. I was so thankful they would be there.

Since she'd first become ill, Elizabeth had watched Sarah unselfishly convert her senior year high school festivities into hospital visitation with only a little time left to celebrate. Sarah had been very much overlooked. Even in all her pain, Elizabeth wrote us a note telling us she wanted all of us focusing only on Sarah on her graduation day.

"I don't want anyone besides John and Tami to visit me that day" she wrote. "I insist!"

In her late afternoon "off the ventilator" session that day, Elizabeth did great. But at one point she grew tired and tried to contact the respiratory therapist to ask him to put her back on the ventilator. She called and no one came. There must have been a lot of critical needs in ICU at that time. She kept trying to get someone to come help her, but still no one came. By the time they actually came, she'd been off the ventilator for six and a half hours, a quarter of a day.

When I left the hospital that night, I shifted into graduation mode, shutting my mind off to what was going on with Elizabeth, except to pray for her. I had to be Sarah's mom the next day. It would require all my strength.

As Sarah's graduation day began, I remembered Elizabeth's intense pain the day before, but refused to allow myself to think about it. I knew if I gave in to it, I'd ignore Sarah as I'd done so much since our whole ordeal began.

After all of our relatives had settled in at the high school to wait for the ceremony to begin, I tried hard to stay focused on the graduation, but my mind kept going back to Elizabeth and her pain. I'd quickly pray for her and put her out of my mind.

"She's in God's hands," I reminded myself. "John and Tami are there. God will use them to help her. Diane, you must mentally remain here at the graduation."

Still, my mind wandered back to Elizabeth. When it did, I started to pinch my arm to remind myself to quickly refocus on Sarah. I thought a small bruise would form on my arm from all the pinching.

"You will enjoy the pride you feel as you see Sarah graduate," I reiterated to myself.

As I tried to exhale calmly and relax, I noticed it really was a beautiful day for a graduation.

Meanwhile, back at the hospital, John and Tami walked into Elizabeth's room with a loving greeting. Elizabeth's downcast face revealed her deep discouragement.

"What's wrong?" asked John.

"I've been in the hospital for such a long time!" she said sadly. "A few weeks ago, I set a goal for myself to attend Sarah's graduation."

"And you didn't get to go," said Tami, as she moved closer to Elizabeth to hear her story.

Tears began falling down Elizabeth's cheeks. John took her hand and tried to comfort her.

"I asked God to get me off the ventilator and out of the hospital by this day," she sobbed. "But He didn't. I'd rather die than be on a ventilator for the rest of my life! I'm never going to get off this ventilator—it's just never going to happen, ever!"

"I can see why you'd feel discouraged," said Tami.

Not long after her heartbreaking confession, Elizabeth began complaining that her lower left lung hurt tremendously. She said it hurt both inhaling and exhaling. The nurse gave her a shot of morphine, which worked for about five minutes. Then they tried a new medicine, which didn't work at all.

John was very tired that morning as well. He sat in a chair near Elizabeth and kept trying to help, but he felt he couldn't since she was so depressed.

"Why am I here?" John wondered. "I'm absolutely exhausted!"

Later that morning, Elizabeth tried pushing through pain as she exercised with the physical therapists. It was difficult for Tami and John to see her in such unrelenting pain.

Tami was sure only God and His resources could enable them to get through the day. She knew they had to pray and read the Word. It was their only hope since it was fact-based, and those facts never change. So Tami tried to get Elizabeth and John to turn their eyes toward Jesus.

"John, do you have a verse for Elizabeth?" she asked.

"No," answered John.

"Elizabeth, do you have a verse for John?" Tami said.

Elizabeth picked up her Bible and lazily flopped a limp hand on the cover without opening it. She didn't have one, either.

"I'll find one for you to give to John, Elizabeth," Tami said.

> "For our light and momentary troubles are achieving for us an eternal glory that far outweighs them all" (2 Corinthians 4:17).

After reading the verse, she gave them a helpful reminder.

"At this very time, your faith is being increased," said Tami. "This faith is the greatest treasure one can have. It is forged through times of doubt."

Their day continued on as it had begun. Elizabeth stared down large quantities of pain and despair.

"Elizabeth looked so bad, I wondered if she was going backwards," Tami said later. "I watched Elizabeth and John have an 'I can't take it anymore' day."

Back in graduation mode, we returned home after Sarah's ceremony for a family celebration. John returned from the hospital just as relatives were starting to leave. He looked quite worn. I could tell by looking at his face that it had been a pretty hard day.

Most of us were sitting in the living room. After a while, grief over Elizabeth's absence that day overwhelmed Sarah. She came in and laid down on the floor.

"I just want my sister back!" she said.

She buried her head in her arms and started to cry.

Matt and I immediately moved to the floor close to her, rubbed her back, and hugged her. She'd said what we were all feeling.

The next morning, I took my parents in to see Elizabeth. They hadn't seen her in over a month. They reveled in all the "first time in a long time" abilities she demonstrated. The Passy-Muir Valve was attached, and they were excited to hear her voice again, too.

Shortly after our arrival, the weekend doctor came in. Elizabeth's grandparents chitchatted with him for a bit, and then their focus turned back to their granddaughter. They asked about her lungs and the ventilator work, and he gave them a thorough update.

"The doctors have differing viewpoints about percentages, but at this point, I think she'll probably end up with 95% lung capacity in her right lung, and 75% in her left," he said. "The doctors feel that's the best they can get them. They don't think that last 30% or so is recoverable. Since her lungs have collapsed so much, they will scar that way and then the scarred portion will eventually fill up with fluid."

"That sounds pretty good, considering what she's been through," said my dad.

"Yes, she was quite sick!" the doctor said.

The doctor had a couple more improvements to mention.

"The leaks in her lungs have healed up, which helps them improve in general," he added. "And just yesterday, they were able to remove one of the chest tubes—that's also a good thing."

Next my parents enthusiastically mentioned her increasing ability to stay off the ventilator some of the time.

"The fact that she's tolerating any time off the ventilator at all is great," the doctor replied. "We were all worried she wouldn't come off it!"

When I heard those words, my protective mother radar shot up.

"Wow—I can't believe he just made such a discouraging comment in front of Elizabeth!" I thought.

By then, I'd fielded and diverted many negative, fearful, or devastating comments from Elizabeth's ears, but I was unable to stop that one—it came out so quickly and unexpectedly. Even though we'd recently begun to be honest with her about what was happening medically, we generally tried to avoid making hopeless, careless remarks.

Elizabeth didn't react when she heard his comment.

I quickly skipped over it and brought up other topics we could pleasantly discuss. Elizabeth and her grandparents had a happy visit. But within an hour or so of their departure, she began to cry.

"Elizabeth, what's the matter?" I asked.

"It's nothing," she said.

She didn't seem to want to talk about it. Family members attempted to comfort her and she seemed okay for a while.

But when tears came again later, I wanted to find out what was troubling her.

"Elizabeth, why are you crying?" I asked. "Is it the doctor's earlier comment?"

"Yes," she said.

"I thought that might be it," I said. "I sure wish he hadn't said that. You shouldn't take his opinion too seriously. That particular doctor really hasn't been involved in much of anything substantial through the course of your illness."

The majority of respiratory therapists, nurses, and doctors had recently been giving her encouraging comments. Sometimes one of her doctors would come in, briefly listen to her lungs with a stethoscope and say, "Excellent!"—that comment carried us all a long way.

We reminded her of comments like that and hoped the negative one would fade away. However, getting one substantially negative comment out of her mind took quite a while.

The next week, during occasional, unhurried moments, Elizabeth and I began to have specific daydreams. Some of hers were just about having the ability to do the many simple daily tasks healthy people take for granted. Another one was to be back at school seeing friends she knew would be overjoyed to see her there.

I had a daydream of Elizabeth entering the circle parking area in front of the main hospital doors and getting into our car to go home. Every day I'd left that exit without her, aching for our final departure together. I'd watched many other happy people do that every day. I couldn't imagine how good that would feel!

One time during Elizabeth's illness I visited The Grant Park Cross, renamed Serra Cross Park in Ventura. The beautiful little park is way up high on a hill and it gives a panoramic view of the Pacific Ocean and its exquisite shoreline for miles. A huge wooden cross stands boldly on top of the hill. I always feel close to God there. During her ICU stay, I also had a daydream of a healthy, ventilator-free Elizabeth standing in that little park with me.

All of her progress meant Elizabeth was able to start using the bedside commode again. Usually when she got out of bed or moved at all, she had two nurses or physical therapists at the same time to help her. But one afternoon, there were many simultaneous needs to be met in ICU. Because the nurses were so busy, Elizabeth had just one nurse helping her in and out of bed.

Whenever Elizabeth needed that type of privacy, we were kept out in the waiting room. We'd been sitting there for an extra long time and didn't know why. Finally, her nurse came out to explain.

"A chest tube was accidentally yanked out and Elizabeth is quite upset about it," she said.

Anger and frustration washed over me after the nurse left.

"How could this have happened?" I asked myself. "I can't bear to think of needless extra pain for Elizabeth. She may have to re-do procedures and wait even longer now because of human error."

It weighed my spirit down. In my heart, I began resenting the person who made the mistake. God knew I especially disliked people hurting my daughters. He kept trying to whittle away my tendency toward harsh reactions whenever human weakness or failure caused unnecessary suffering or deterioration. But I couldn't let it go.

Two friends came by for a visit and one handed me words from the hymn "He Giveth More Grace" she'd copied on a 4 x 6 card. I needed them just about then:

"He giveth more grace when our burdens grow greater
He sendeth more strength as our labors increase;
To added afflictions He addeth His mercy
To multiplied trials His multiplied peace
    When we have exhausted our store of endurance
    When our strength has failed ere the day is half done
    When we reach the end of our hoarded resources
    Our Father's full giving is only begun
Chorus
His love has no limits, His grace has no measure
His power no boundary known unto men
For out of His infinite riches in Jesus
He giveth and giveth and giveth again."[14]

My mind tried to assimilate those glorious truths. They eased me away from my anger some.

When we returned to Elizabeth's room later, I could tell she'd been crying and that her nurse had worked hard to calm her down. I knew it wouldn't do any good to say anything about it just then, so I didn't.

The doctor discovered that the tube that had been pulled out from her left lung had been water sealed and just left in place for a week or so.

"There wasn't a better tube for that to happen to, since it was almost ready to be removed," he said. "It caused no new problem."

"God had her back," I thought.

---

14   "He Giveth More Grace," words by Annie Johnson Flint, Printed at Orchard Park, NY in "Casterline Card" Series, Public Domain.

Before leaving for the night, we learned how the chest tube was yanked out. Elizabeth had been ready to return to bed, but the tubing that went from her chest to each individual monitoring box was not carefully moved out of her way. As she stood up, Elizabeth herself accidentally stepped on the chest tube, painfully yanking it out of her own chest. The site began bleeding excessively.

The nurse didn't notice at first. Elizabeth couldn't speak because the PMV wasn't attached then, so she made a huge, silent "Owwwww!" face repeatedly and waved her arms frantically to get her nurse's attention.

Once alerted, the nurse began doing damage control.

"So much for resenting the person who made the mistake!" I thought, briefly loathing myself.

Even though she was weak and tired from a recent illness, and she'd had an upsetting afternoon, substantial ventilator weaning progress was taking place. She had an off-the-ventilator session that evening which lasted close to nine hours. She was still trying to move forward. When we went into her room for our final evening visit, she was smiling.

Because of Matt's return to work full time during the week, we began functioning more like a tag-team as we visited and supported our daughter. Even so, in our brief times together, I noticed another subtle shift in our marriage had taken place. Matt didn't react emotionally to new developments like I did. He persevered well. He'd learned to lean fully on God and one of the benefits was that I could lean more on him.

The next morning, I began my day feeling down. I was alone in the waiting room expecting to be buzzed inside ICU soon. I looked out the window. The view and my heart were both dreary. I knew what I should do, but I didn't feel like doing it. I could have turned to God's Word and claimed a Psalm, maybe one like Psalm 4:1.

> "Answer me when I call to You, O my righteous God.
> Give me relief from my distress; be merciful to me and hear my prayer."

But I didn't. Uncertainty hung heavily on me and I asked myself some questions.

"Will Elizabeth ever get off the ventilator? What will her life be like if she doesn't? How and when will this all end? How many more days will I be in this room looking out at a gloomy, overcast sky?"

No one had the answers to my tough questions except God, and He was keeping me in a waiting, faith-growing silence.

Inside ICU, Elizabeth woke up with a 102-degree fever, an extremely achy body, and nausea. It looked like stomach flu. She felt utterly terrible and was 99% unwilling to move because she felt so bad. Being sick again was getting very old.

As I went through those months with my daughter, I learned that suffering was one thing, but longsuffering was quite another. Longsuffering has been defined as "enduring trouble, pain, or injury long and patiently." As I sat beside her bed that day, I witnessed true longsuffering.

Elizabeth still felt terrible when I returned from a lunch break. I hated seeing her that way. Her nurse tried to get her to move to do physical therapy, but she had little luck. Elizabeth's body needed another resting day, and she was going to take it!

I had to fight my urges to pick her up and race to the hospital exit with her. I sat beside her bed, full of dark thoughts.

"I feel like I'm sitting in quick-drying cement," I moaned inwardly. "It seems like I'll be here forever."

My gloomy outlook intensified.

"Will we ever leave this place?" I wondered.

CHAPTER SEVENTEEN

Plans for a Hope and a Future

ELIZABETH'S FEVERS AND NEW INFECTIONS grew in intensity and frequency the following week. She ran a fever four out of seven days. Even in her misery, forward progress was made through chest tube therapy. Another chest tube was removed and settings were adjusted to put the three remaining tubes on water seal. A couple of days later, the chest tube doctor returned to remove one more tube—three down, only two to go.

In addition, Elizabeth had big news for us when we entered her room one morning that week—she'd stayed off the ventilator comfortably for a total of eleven hours during the previous 24 hour period. Hope began to return.

Within a couple more days, the flu bug had officially passed and she felt somewhat stronger. Her physical therapists arrived and prepared her for a walk. Since the remaining two chest tubes were water sealed, it meant mobility and freedom had finally been achieved! Elizabeth was no longer dependent on suction. She could walk out of her room or go anywhere for a short time using a small, portable canister of oxygen.

Soon she was out of her bed and standing steadily. They headed her toward the door and picked up her chest tube monitor boxes. Elizabeth walked out of her ICU room, #19, for the first time, all the way down to the doorway of room #15, with one physical therapist walking closely beside her on either side.

Her walk through ICU was a good stretch for her. Smiles beamed from every thrilled face on the hospital staff as she walked by them!

I walked behind her and noticed the sweet, familiar sound of her left toe popping. I cherished even that simple piece of evidence that Elizabeth was coming back to us.

Many substantial improvements were occurring simultaneously, and they all moved her closer to being weaned off the ventilator. The following morning Elizabeth reported staying off the ventilator for 16 ½ hours.

"You'll be able to go through the night before you know it!" said her respiratory therapist.

Elizabeth's newfound mobility and freedom sparked the idea of taking her outside for a wheelchair ride. Great enthusiasm accompanied plans that were in the making for this event. Every available family member plus John got in on it.

Sarah missed the first outing but she was thrilled when it was her turn to take her sister outside.

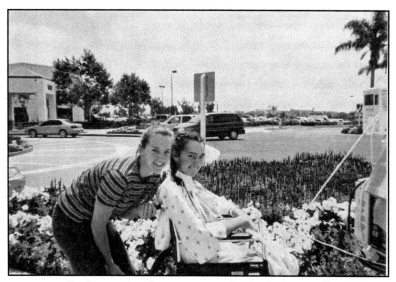

Sarah stopping for a picture with Elizabeth outside

Our Ever-Present Help

By her sixth week of chest tube therapy, her doctors really wanted to get her out of the hospital sooner rather than later because of the recurrent hospital-acquired infections. As they discussed future plans for Elizabeth, we heard wonderful phrases like: "before she goes home," "home is best," and "going home is imminent within the next week or two." Our hearts leapt for joy when we heard the word "home."

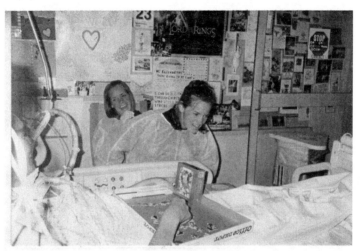

Elizabeth works a puzzle in bed while Maggie and Sarah share excitement about her coming home prospects

Before leaving, we wanted a picture of Elizabeth and her primary doctor.

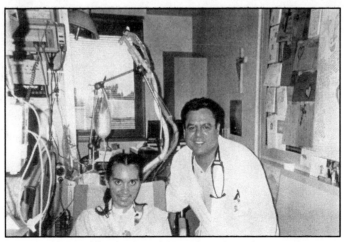

Elizabeth and Dr. Glen Abergel

After much discussion, they planned to send her to a regular room on the second floor for about a week and then home. The last piece of information we needed was—when?

We were happy enough to hear the word "home." But all along Elizabeth's journey toward recovery, we couldn't help ourselves. We had to celebrate each significant "first." Her first chocolate shake since before her illness was special as were her first family hugs.

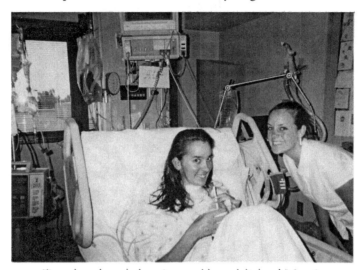

First chocolate shake witnessed by a delighted Maggie

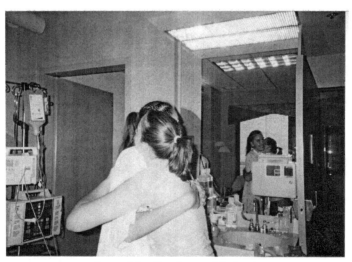

One of the first hugs with Sarah

From time to time on our journey with Elizabeth, I noticed behaving normally in social situations had begun to elude me. Acting awkward, weird and just plain strange at times became my new "normal." It was apparent that day when three Bible study friends, Joy, Susan, and Mary, took me to lunch. It felt so good to be with them. We got Chinese food and while we ate, I began to update them on possible going home plans for Elizabeth.

I'd loaded up my fork with fried rice to eat it, but while I was talking, I put my fork back down and dug it into the clump of rice on my plate. I left the fork handle extended off the edge of the plate near my right hand. As I finished making my point, I made a hand gesture. Without thinking about the placement of my fork handle, I suddenly brought my right hand down. It hit the fork handle, pushing it down quickly.

A large load of rice was catapulted into the air. It went straight up over my head and began landing all over the table, my hair, clothes, and the floor. It felt like heavy rain. It seemed to go everywhere. I was shocked at how much rice I'd spread all around me and my place at the table. My friends were very surprised. I began to worry about myself.

I cleaned up as much as I could and we finished our lunch. Mary drove me back to the hospital entrance. As I got out, I saw a few pieces of rice that I'd carried and deposited on the floor of her car.

"Pick up your rice and go," said Mary, laughing.

So, I did.

About an hour later, back in Elizabeth's room, I happened to look down toward my feet. I noticed a few more pieces of rice lying inside the top edges of my socks. I dug the rice out and threw it away. Lunch was officially over.

When I walked into ICU the next morning, I was very eager to see how long Elizabeth had stayed off the ventilator through the night.

"How did your night go?" I asked.

"I stayed off the ventilator all night, and I feel comfortable!" she reported with great delight. "I'm still off the ventilator now!"

That news took my own breath away! My spirit bowed right then and there before my God who'd enabled this mighty thing. I was speechless.

Then I suddenly became aware of an astounding fact.

"I've walked into 'Miracle Territory'. I'm looking at and talking to a true miracle of God!"

Then my words returned to me.

"She did it!!!!!" I exclaimed. "Oh, Lord, she did it! Thank you, Lord!"

It was invigorating for everyone to see the impossible happen! Her room was suddenly packed with joy and smiles.

Elizabeth's "day" had finally come and Dr. Abergel knew it.

"This is all very encouraging," he said. "I'm very pleased! She's moving in the right direction. Home is near. When she goes three to four nights off the ventilator without realizing it, they can get rid of it."

"For once, I didn't miss a great doctor report!" I thought as I laughed out loud.

Word spread quickly through the hospital staff that Elizabeth had stayed off the ventilator all night and remained off. Elated medical personnel stopped by briefly from various places in the hospital to join the joyful hubbub. They smiled broadly and made enthusiastic comments.

Even the thoracic surgeon seemed delighted.

"I wouldn't have believed it if I didn't see it!" He remarked.

When Matt arrived hours later, I pointed out the miracle. He felt deeply thankful.

I still couldn't believe my own eyes and ears. Her success and the joy it generated were abundantly good!

Later that afternoon, I sat quietly for a while in Elizabeth's room thinking about the people who'd prayed for her. Back in April, they each believed God could do exactly what we saw that day in June. Her restored abilities to breathe were empowered by energy from the living God poured out on her behalf over a two and a half month period. I'm sure He was smiling as He watched her lovely breathing.

What an extraordinary day! Miracle Territory continued glowing with wonder as daylight faded into darkness!

"Let everything that has breath praise the Lord. Praise the Lord" (Psalm 150:6).

One day after the next, Elizabeth stayed off the ventilator. We slowly got used to seeing that beautiful, miraculous occurrence. I loved it every time I saw it! God was so good! Those were exciting days.

Then, one afternoon, a respiratory therapist entered her room, moved a few things to clear a path, and suddenly wheeled out her ventilator. Just like that, it was gone! Awesome. *Praise God!*

"Now that's what I'm talking about!" I cried out.

As Elizabeth drew near to the time she'd leave ICU, it was easy to see that Matt had continued to grow spiritually. Changes were becoming permanent. It was hard to tell all the exact measures used in that process. In her book, *Come Away My Beloved*, Frances J. Roberts relates God's explanation of one of His most powerful yet mysterious methods for creating spiritual growth. It was probably a part of the mix for Matt.

> "Be occupied with acquainting yourself with My character and My person. Revel in My fellowship. Your very association with Me, if sufficiently consistent, will bring about changes in your personality that will surprise you when discovered; just as you have so often experienced the joy of finding a new bloom on a cherished plant."

She goes on further to describe one of the Lord's reasons for wanting believers to delight themselves in Him.

> "In association with others, people take to themselves a measure of the mannerisms and ideologies of these other persons. So will it be for those who spend much time in My company.
> Silently, and without conscious effort, you will be changed."[15]

My daughters and I saw the results of the Lord's ongoing personality makeover in Matt. He was more yielded, submissive, and devoted to God. A new kind of joy showed on his face. His heart change was evident by the words that came out of his mouth.

---

15 Frances J. Roberts, <u>Come Away My Beloved</u>, #220-221, © 1970. Material is being used by permission of Barbour Publishing, Inc., Uhrichsville, Ohio.

Elizabeth and I noticed it one morning when Matt and I happened to be in her room together. She was to move out of ICU that day, so we started taking down the many get well cards and pictures sent by loved ones that had decorated her Oxnard hospital home.

One particular card caught Matt's eye as he worked. He read it again. It had come earlier when Elizabeth's struggle had been most intense. On the cover it showed a weak, exhausted man with anguish on his face. His knees were buckling and he was about to fall, but Jesus was also in the picture. His face was full of compassion as He lovingly reached around from behind to take hold of the man and keep him from falling. It was a beautiful picture of Jesus' powerful, helping embrace. Inside the card was a reminder to Elizabeth that Jesus was carrying her.

"The truth shown in this card is beautiful," he said.

It continued to amaze me to hear Matt initiate a conversation about the goodness of his God.

As Elizabeth adjusted to being in a regular room, she realized how much the medical team in ICU had kept her physically active. In her new room, the "pushers" were gone.

However, one afternoon, Dr. Abergel showed up and made the way for another joyful walk outside with Elizabeth. The three of us had a glorious time in the fresh air and sunshine.

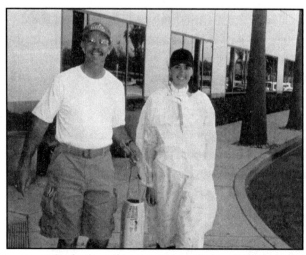

Elizabeth walking outside with her father

Even though non-motivation set in easily in her regular room, one thing in particular highly motivated Elizabeth as the exit door drew near. She really wanted to return to Biola to finish her final semester and graduate in December. She called the registration office at Biola to get the ball rolling. She hoped to start the very next semester, which was about six weeks away. The person she spoke with told her someone at the school had already pre-registered her for the classes she dropped in the spring. After a series of calls, her complete schedule was set for the fall semester.

I felt uncertainty about whether she could handle her plan. I thought she might be rushing it. But then I remembered the Bible verse that had been sent to her from family and friends most often during her illness.

> "For I know the plans I have for you," declares the Lord,
> "plans to prosper you and not to harm you, plans to give
> you a hope and a future" (Jeremiah 29:11).

The excited, confident look on my daughter's face was priceless. Elizabeth already saw plans for her future unfolding. Whenever people called or came by, she confidently and happily told them she was going back to Biola.

It was as if the Lord put His stamp of approval on her life as she came to the end of her illness and suffering. A psalm puts it in the following way:

> "He brought me out into a spacious place; He rescued me
> because He delighted in me" (Psalm 18:19).

I saw I needed to get out of the way of her faith and her heart.

The next day, Elizabeth was given a quilt handmade by a family friend, Gayle Moyer. From the beginning to the end of her journey, Elizabeth had been beautifully wrapped up in the loving arms of the Body of Christ.

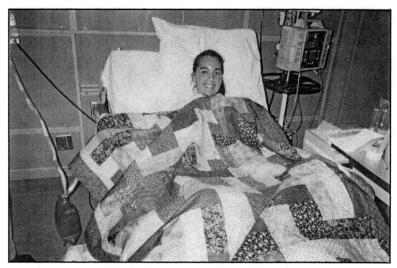

Elizabeth covered with Gayle's quilt

One doctor after another stopped by during her final week to give concluding recommendations and well wishes to Elizabeth. Her remaining tubes were removed without incident.

Then on July 16—94 days after I first drove with her to the emergency room—her family was ready to take her home.

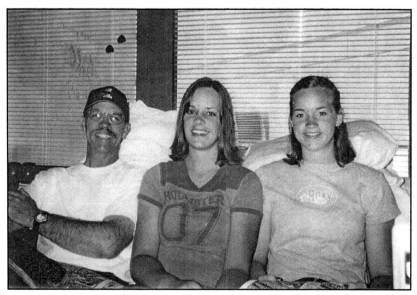

Matt, Maggie, and Sarah eagerly awaiting Elizabeth's release from the hospital

We waited all morning for her to be discharged. We had a Subway sandwich picnic lunch in her hospital room. We waited through the afternoon and still no one came to discharge her. Sarah had to go to work. We began to wonder if it would happen that day after all.

Finally, that evening—her discharge papers were signed and she was released. Hallelujah!!!

At 7:00 p.m. Elizabeth began her "just discharged" wheelchair ride down the main hospital entrance. At last! It was glorious! She sat down in our van. We were ready to go.

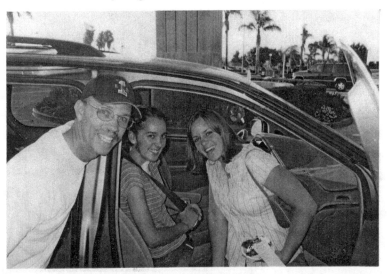

"She's in our car! Let's go!"

We had a happy freeway drive toward home. Matt and Maggie drove in separate cars and we waved, honked from car to car, and shared gigantic smiles through our windows. Sarah was very disappointed she couldn't be with us.

Elizabeth seemed so glad to see everything around her. She'd been gone so long. After walking into the house, she lovingly greeted our dog with a "Hi, Ruffy!" and petted him briefly. Then she sat on our couch. Her every movement held us spellbound.

She was finally home and relaxing. It felt wonderful! Our spirits soared!

As soon as her shift was over, Sarah quickly drove home and ran into the house to give Elizabeth a warm, loving, "welcome home" hug. It was so good to have the entire family home together again!

<hr />

The news "Elizabeth is home!" stirred people everywhere her story was known. One woman immediately cried big puddles of joyful, thankful tears when she read an e-mail proclaiming the news. Another wiped away happy tears that came intermittently after she heard. Once Elizabeth was out and about, people who knew her just stopped and stared when they saw her. Shocked looks of disbelief were a normal occurrence in church when this miracle walked in and sat down in their midst. Those were good times!

But the main thing that continued stirring Elizabeth was returning to Biola. Her heart was set on it. During her five weeks of recovery time at home, she and Maggie made plans to share a dorm room at Biola. Maggie quickly transferred from APU to Biola, and just before the fall semester began, they moved back to school again.

When Elizabeth first arrived at Biola, she began seeing friends everywhere she went. Much like people at home, they were astounded to see her. They could barely believe their eyes. Some screamed joyfully when they first saw her. Others responded with their mouths dropping open in astonishment. Each amazed reaction revealed their overwhelming wonder at what God had done.

<hr />

Once Elizabeth and Maggie settled in at Biola, things slowed down a little at home. I took some time to write a thank you letter to the elders of our church. It read:

"When our daughter, Elizabeth, suddenly became critically ill in mid-April, my husband, family, and I were so thankful you gathered so quickly that first night to anoint her head with oil and pray for God to heal her. The sight of holy men of God gathering and uniting in His Spirit in the face of something that appeared humanly impossible was precious.

In those early days and weeks, we wanted to let you know how much we appreciated your prayer support on so many occasions. Most of you came on that first Monday night. Some also came later that week on

Thursday night when septic shock became a serious threat. Many of you came by, sent cards, and reassured us regularly of your continuing prayers on her behalf. Still others came to pray with us again weeks later when our burden grew heavier in Oxnard. I said we *wanted* to thank you, but we never really did. The right time never seemed to come since weeks turned into months.

The Lord did many miracles as He healed our daughter. So many times she'd get to one place and stay there. Then, as God's people prayed on, He moved her to the next phase of healing. We know God had His reasons for all He allowed and for each phase of timing.

In a recent quiet time, I was reading in Matthew 8 and 9. These two chapters tell many stories of Jesus healing people of various infirmities or illnesses. God pointed out some beautiful truths to me as I meditated on them. In one story, Jesus healed a leper. It seemed important in that story that Jesus was *willing* to heal him. He proved that He was. Another time Jesus wanted people to believe He was *able* to heal. And in other situations, Jesus said He healed *according to their faith*. In Elizabeth's case, all three of these elements were present.

As we all prayed for God's will in her healing, the first thing we knew was that Jesus was able to heal. Next we prayed that Jesus was willing to heal her. He proved that He was. And lastly, we saw Him respond to the faith demonstrated in fervent, believing prayer. Willing, able, and according to faith. God enabled and performed it all. He is to be fully praised for all He has done. Thanks so much for being an invaluable part of this miraculous story.

Our entire family thanks you so much for ministering to each of us wholeheartedly and with excellence in the name of Jesus. We've seen wondrous things and we're overflowing with gratitude. We've truly been blessed.

In the name of our wonder-working God, The McGovern Family

A month and a half after Elizabeth returned to Biola, Matt and I took a walk along the shoreline of a secluded beach one day. I was still processing what we'd just been through. While we walked, I saw a perfect picture of one of God's resources that had helped us through our recent crisis.

As we went farther down the beach, I noticed groups of small, ordinary-looking gray birds digging for sand crabs as waves came and went. Matt said he thought they were sandpipers. They seemed to have an "avoid the water" rule, which they all followed, even though they were comfortable at its very edge. As I watched them, I noticed their repetitive pattern. They'd accompany a receding wave down to the edge of the water to dig for their desired food. They had only seconds to eat before the next wave came. Then, when it broke, they'd race up to the shore outrunning the breaking wave. Their tiny legs moved so fast, I couldn't focus clearly on them. Their movements were rapid, accurate, perfectly timed, and purposeful.

We continued walking near them while they ate. They eventually sensed we were getting too close and seemed to feel threatened. They all suddenly flew away from us, putting a safe distance between us and them. As they took to flight, their wing spans opened up revealing their most beautiful physical feature—black wings with a striking white stripe in the middle. These dull-colored, gray birds became most beautiful when they felt threatened. Under calm, normal circumstances, their beauty was hidden.

These little birds reminded me of the Body of Christ during Elizabeth's illness. While her life was threatened, believers functioned rapidly and purposefully to minister to her and our family any way they could. As God drew all of us together to face that threat, the faith, love, hope, comfort, and support of the faithful ones who drew near was attractive to all who saw it. The little gray birds weren't much to look at until they responded together to a threat in their territory, and neither is the Body of Christ.

In scripture, the Lord through Paul teaches believers how to act as members of His body.

> "Be devoted to one another in brotherly love. Honor one another above yourselves. Never be lacking in zeal, but keep your spiritual fervor, serving the Lord. Be joyful in hope, patient in affliction, faithful in prayer. Share with God's people who are in need. Practice hospitality" (Romans 12:10–13 NASB).

We witnessed these strikingly beautiful godly behaviors up close. Through His people, God took such good care of us during our time of trouble.

A couple of months into the Fall school semester, Matt and I attended another parent visitation weekend at Biola. On Friday afternoon we'd arranged to meet Maggie, John and Elizabeth for lunch. Maggie and John found us first.

Then I saw Elizabeth coming around the bend in the road, swinging her skinny arms and throwing her weight into those still recovering legs. Her head was held high. I looked at her determined young face. It was a fact—she loved being back at Biola! I knew she loved her God with all her strength. She knew His power and goodness. Admiration for my courageous, faithful daughter filled my being.

"That girl is something else!" I said.

CHAPTER EIGHTEEN

Testify

IN OCTOBER 2004, GOD GAVE Elizabeth the opportunity to share her testimony at Biola on their Day of Prayer. She was introduced by Ron Hafer, the Chaplain.

"When I was a student here at Talbot Seminary hundreds of years ago, they said, 'If you have an illustration, make it be a powerful one in keeping with the text,' he said. "The text is prayer and what our awesome God can do and the illustration is the story that Elizabeth McGovern is going to share. This is a huge story and this is her first opportunity before the student body. It's a limited time to tell a great story of God's grace. Last semester, we were praying that God would keep her alive for another 24-hour period. He's done far more than that."

Then my brave daughter stepped behind the podium and gave her testimony:

"It's *so good* to be here and I want to say that God is *so good*.

"Last semester during spring break, I went home and I was kind of sick. I ended up going to the hospital. I had viral pneumonia in both my lungs and things got worse and worse while I was there. Like Ron said, there was one day, actually there were a few days, where it looked like I wouldn't even make it or be alive the next day. But God did amazing things.

"Both my lungs collapsed. The doctors told my parents I had about a 50% chance of living. And then, something else went wrong and it became, 'maybe a 40% chance.' And then things kept getting worse and they stopped telling them the percentage, because I wasn't supposed to live. But God had other plans. He was working all of the time in everything. When things started getting really bad, my parents asked some people to pray for me.

"And God raised a *huge* prayer support team. A lot of you probably prayed for me. People from different churches prayed. Many from a former church where my parents were married 25 years ago prayed. So did some in other states and even other countries. There was one grandmother of a Biola student that I didn't even know who prayed faithfully. It was amazing. God drew so many people in to pray for me. It was nothing we did. It was totally God.

"I was unconscious for nine days in the hospital, and when I woke up, it was scary and lonely. I wasn't breathing on my own. A machine breathed for me, and I had things feeding me. I felt really alone and I was in a lot of pain physically. I felt really out of it for the first few weeks after I woke up.

"During that time, I also wasn't able to talk because of the big tube in my mouth and throat. I couldn't write because I'd become really weak and my muscles had turned to noodles.

"But during that time, I felt like the Lord was right there with me and He just held me in His arms. He'd speak to me.

Elizabeth, I'm here with you.

"Time and time again, I'd feel overwhelmed.

'Oh, my gosh, I can't do this, I can't do this!' I'd think.

"But He'd remind me of His presence.

Elizabeth, I'm here. Elizabeth, trust Me. It will be okay.

"He brought so many people around to visit me. My family was there almost every day. My boyfriend came so much. A lot of my friends as well as people from church came to see me, too. God used them to bring me joy whether they held my hand, told a joke, made a funny face, prayed with me, sang songs, or braided my hair. God used so many people to support and encourage me, and I'm so thankful for them. I have a stack of cards about this big (motioned 2–3" distance with finger and thumb) from people who sent me cards and said they were praying for me.

"There were hard days, but God always brought something to remind me that He was there and He was good. One day I was having a bad day and a bad attitude. I had to get another x-ray—I got x-rays a lot. And this new guy came in with a big smile. He was quite short and somewhat older. He was so cute.

'Hi, Elizabeth!' he said. 'How are you today?'

"Huh," I moaned. 'I'm all right.'

"Something prompted him to ask if I was a Christian. I nodded my head and he gave me a huge smile again. He enthusiastically told me he was too, and that he'd pray for me.

"God, you're so cool," I thought. This guy I don't even know was so sweet to me. And he's praying for me, you know."

"And through all that prayer, through everything, God did so many miracles. I was supposed to die. I went and had a checkup after I got out of the hospital.

'We normally study cases like yours in an autopsy room,' said the doctor.

'Wow!" I thought.

"It is an amazing testimony to God that He's powerful and He still does miracles. I might have needed a lung transplant at one point, but I didn't. I might have remained on the machine for the rest of my life, but God had other plans.

No, you're going to get better.

"I might not have been able to talk ever again, but, obviously, I can talk.

"And when God brought me home to my house and my family, it was a miracle. I was in the hospital for three months and two days. The day after I got home, I had a really special time with my family and my boyfriend. We had a time of reflection and shared comments.

'God, You are so good!'

'You did so much!'

'Thank You for saving me.'

'Thank You for bringing us ALL through this hard time!'

"I have a verse I picked out that I like.

> 'Unless the Lord had given me hope, I would soon have dwelt in the silence of death. When I said "my foot is slipping," Your love, oh, Lord, supported me. When

anxiety was great within me, your consolation brought joy to my soul' (Psalm 94:17–19).

"You probably won't have the same thing happen to you that happened to me. But I just wanted to encourage you, that when you're going through hard times, God's there with you. He's there, and He knows what you're going through. Just keep praying. Take your *huge* requests to Him because He answers them. He always has the best in mind for us.

"I was thinking about everything I went through, and I wouldn't trade it for anything. God taught me so much. Even though it was a horrible situation, God was good. God brought me out of it and taught me patience. He comforted me and He gave me joy and peace. And He can do the same thing for you."

―

Elizabeth and John were busy with normal, healthy life in many ways. God Himself was establishing them after they'd suffered together. As a matter of fact, they became engaged two months after her graduation.

Eight months later, on October 15, 2005, Elizabeth walked down a daisy-studded path toward the man of her dreams on their wedding day. The day, the outdoor setting, and the couple were beautiful. God brought family and friends from near and far. It was a godly, worshipful ceremony, much like I pictured in my daydream way back in April 2004. Elizabeth even chose to have a string quartet play Pachelbel's *Canon in D Major* while her bridesmaids walked down the aisle.

We all rejoiced over His hand upon John and Elizabeth as He blessed their marriage. Tears came once again when I saw my daughter in that setting after almost losing her. We stood amazed.

On the wedding invitation, they printed: "How can I repay the Lord for all His goodness to me?" from Psalm 116:12.

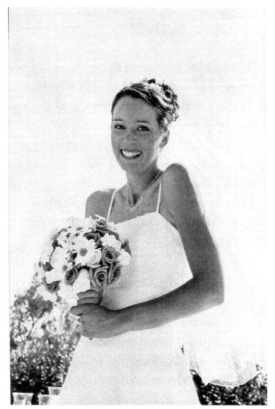

An overjoyed Elizabeth on her wedding day

♥ ♥ ♥ ♥ ♥ ♥ ♥ ♥ ♥ ♥

When Elizabeth first came home from the hospital, I found myself in a place I'd never been before. I thought back to the way things had been before her illness. My husband and I had turned our parental control knobs off when she left for college. But during her health crisis we quickly turned them to the highest level. After three months on "high" concern, my knob had broken off, but the control level remained on "high." I couldn't figure out how to turn it back off.

For some reason, it took me a while to believe she was well. I struggled with the adjustment between Elizabeth's two extreme health categories: "terribly sick" and "well." No one else in my family had the same problem. Since Elizabeth got well, significant things had been happening in all of their lives. Even after the crisis was over, God still had another important faith lesson for me to learn.

During her first days at home, many positive emotions were stirred when we saw Elizabeth everywhere in our house again. We were so blessed by God. But one emotion came completely unexpectedly and began to dominate me mercilessly—fear. Instead of focusing on the miracle God performed, I began concentrating incorrectly on how easily I could lose a daughter. It surprised me when I faintly saw sin and temptation crouching at my door, desiring to have me.

You must master it, whispered the Holy Spirit.

But I didn't pay attention.

In those early post-hospital days, I was unbelievably tired and felt my faith was utterly spent. I really wanted God to lift His intense gaze off of me for a while. I hoped for a period of smooth sailing. But instead of a relaxing pleasure cruise, I foolishly, unknowingly signed myself up for a journey in a one-man fear boat.

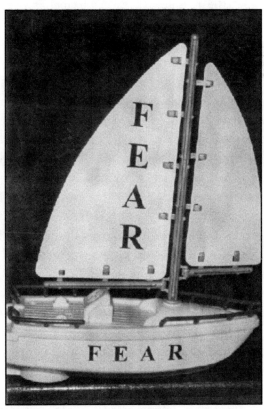

The *Fear Boat*

My boat was destined to take me deep into a world ruled by fear. The Lord didn't want me to go on the journey, but I was too tired to check with Him beforehand. However, my boat would keep me safely afloat for the whole trip, sometimes just barely, because I belonged to Jesus. My life was in Jesus' hands. Even in my sorry state, He'd protect me.

As I began slowly drifting away from the dock of faith and realism, I began feeling afraid of anything that could affect Elizabeth's newly-recovered lungs. If she sat or stood up too long, which caused her to breathe faster, I got edgy. If it was windy when she went outside, I didn't like it. An unexpected stairway for her to navigate made me nervous. If she developed a new cough or fever, a feeling of dread came over me. John took her on a drive an hour away one night and I was fearful. I drifted farther from the dock of faith. I began losing sight of anything familiar.

After two or three months in my fear boat, I made a stink about plans for a possible trip to the mountains because Elizabeth might have breathing problems due to the higher elevation. No one but me felt concerned about it. I discovered one fear bred hundreds more. A repetitive tape of fear thoughts began running through my mind.

Then, almost a year into my fear journey, another significant occasion came along. Matt and I celebrated our 26th wedding anniversary by spending a weekend together in Monterey, California. On Saturday morning, we walked along the coast. We sat for a while on a bench overlooking the breathtaking shoreline. Still in my fear boat, somehow I arranged things so I could sit in my boat and on the bench near my husband at the same time. We relaxed and talked. He knew I still struggled with fear.

"I want God to give me assurance that Elizabeth will have a healthy future," I said. "I want her to be the same as before she got sick."

I had a death grip on her future.

"God won't give you that information," Matt explained. "We have to trust Him and live by faith. She may live a long, healthy life, but God is the only One who knows that."

When I heard mature spiritual advice coming out of Matt, I realized something profound was happening. The Lord was richly blessing us with a lovely, spiritual conversation! I'd shared my vulnerability and immediately received his faith-inspiring comment. It felt so right and good.

In that moment my heart felt well-taken care of and content. Our marriage relationship had deepened so we could also function as a brother and sister in Christ. Sitting on that bench, I realized I was sitting in the place I'd longed for—years before Elizabeth became deathly ill. God is so good!

Yet during those "fear" months, I heard wise encouragement like his, but not long afterwards, something triggered another fear impulse. I quickly forgot wise words and drifted farther away than I was before. It seemed people around me couldn't help me permanently and they got tired of my attitude. I got tired of myself, as well.

I was growing weary of my unrelenting fears yet my rough ride lasted many more months.

"How do I get out of this fear boat?" I began to wonder. "God said He always provides a way of escape when believers are tempted to sin. Where is my way of escape?"

Those who belong to Jesus Christ know the answer. It's always the same answer. Had I turned to Him for help at the beginning when I felt pressured into my fear boat, or anywhere along the journey, He would have pulled me out and kept me safe. It was like He was in a huge, fully loaded Coast Guard vessel just nearby on my ocean of fear. He would have raced to my help if I'd just called Him and really meant it.

Of course, I prayed a little about these fears many times. I prayed polite, simple, passive prayers and asked God to help me. But I still allowed myself a little room to tolerate my fear. My prayers were wishy-washy. I wasn't sincere and I saw no apparent help afterwards. I incorrectly believed a lie—"Even God can't help me!" I felt too lost to trust Him for help.

My mind raged out-of-control.

"What am I doing?" I asked myself. "I've just seen unbelievable miracles!!! How can I be fearful now? This makes no sense! It's ridiculous!"

Yet it went on month after month, even when Elizabeth had no serious problems.

"What if something goes wrong in her lungs again?" I asked myself constantly.

After Elizabeth and John had been married for a few months, my fear boat suffered damage. It hit a big jagged rock just under the surface and a rogue wave was suddenly heading right for me.

John and Elizabeth were preparing to counsel high school students at a winter camp. Elizabeth called and asked me to pray that she'd know whether or not to go, since she had a head cold. I told her I'd pray, but I was definitely the wrong person to ask at that point.

After I got off the phone, I realized fear had become a stronghold in my mind. It was dark, vicious, and relentless. I was deeply tormented. My mind was at war. An immediate fear thought came as I tried to pray about Elizabeth's camp decision.

"She may get sicker in the snow in a higher altitude and that would be very bad for her, maybe even dangerous," I thought. "And there isn't a hospital near the camp."

The next morning Matt called to check on Elizabeth. In my insecurity, I felt that Elizabeth and John didn't want to talk to me because they knew what I'd say. At that point, they knew Matt walked in faith. They could trust him to be reasonable and sensible.

Feeling useless, I wandered back to our bedroom, laid down on the bed and started to cry. Brutal thoughts badgered my mind again and pushed me over the edge. I was sick to death of fear! God moved me to that precious place of desperation where effective prayer and aggressive action finally take place.

That morning, I humbled myself and called to Jesus in my brokenness. I confessed my sin of fear and the grip it had on me. I confessed my absolute helplessness to get free of it. I finally started praying correctly again.

God reminded me that I had to completely reject any tolerance of my sinful fear. I needed to adopt a "No more Mr. Nice Guy!" philosophy toward it. As I continued praying, He led me to pray boldly and ask for His powerful help. I was sure I needed the big guns. I remembered only my God had that kind of power.

Next, God took aggressive action to help me. He took the fear out of my heart and instigated a firm, new plan for me. I kept praying and listening carefully to God.

Now, Diane, you've had such a hard time with this fear. Here's the first part of my plan—I'm going to have to fire you as Elizabeth's health care overseer. This part of your mothering job is over. She's married and her health decisions are no longer yours to make.

Here's what you must do. First, you are not to dwell on one thought about her health. If you do, it's a sin for you. Second, you are never to talk about it anymore with concern and worry. Third, you are to treat her like a normal person again. And last, you can pray to Me to guide John and Elizabeth to make wise decisions about her health needs.

In those precious moments, He quickly pulled my fear boat back to the dock of faith and reality. He got me out of the boat and pointed me toward the shore again. Then He turned and destroyed my fear boat.

God describes His actions perfectly in His Word.

> "He reached down from on high and took hold of me; He drew me out of deep waters. He rescued me from my powerful enemy, from my foes, who were too strong for me. They confronted me in the day of my disaster, but the Lord was my support" (Psalm 18:16–18).

And another psalm mentions His rescue abilities.

> "I sought the Lord, and He answered me; He delivered me from all my fears" (Psalm 34:4).

Shortly after God's work in my heart that day, I began experiencing His goodness again. I felt free from my fear bondage and I had a right mind again. The Lord also renewed my ability to exhibit the fruit of the Holy Spirit.

I tried to analyze why I went on the fear journey. I didn't know that sometimes our spiritual enemy loves to attack God's people mercilessly after any great spiritual victory the Lord has won in their lives. He is the master of cruel surprise attacks. He especially loves to work us over when we're weak.

In my exhaustion, I was ignorant and unobservant. I put myself in a very vulnerable place. I didn't realize I still needed God's spiritual protection. I'd laid down my precious, proven spiritual weapons. I thought I deserved to take a break from my faith walk, and that it would be okay to rely on my own strength for a while.

But, by taking a vacation from God, I opened myself up to worldly solutions to problems that arose. Without realizing it, I left myself open to seek solutions to life's problems elsewhere. Even total self-reliance can be a pit. The world always entices people to follow some "new" spiritual path. In the end, if a believer goes that way, they end up trying to combine these new beliefs with their Christianity—the old hodgepodge idea that sounds good at first but produces nothing but a shipwreck in regards to faith.

Sometimes, even strong believers turn away from the Lord and it's grievous to see. When I tried it, I learned there's no fruitful, happy in-between ground. Throughout all generations, faith and fear have remained mutually exclusive!

If you've wandered off your path with the Lord for any reason, there's hope. Wherever you are and whatever you're going through, you can be sure of this—at any moment you can look up again and seriously reconnect with Him. He wants to send you effective help. He's waiting for you to call on Him. One of the most beautiful prayers to God is a short one—"Help!"

Many people and things in life may let you down, but God never will. Maybe you're facing the worst thing you've ever been through in your life. He is there for you. If you're as low as you've ever been or if you're experiencing utter failure, He is there. Maybe you can honestly say the bottom has dropped out of your life. He's underneath you to catch you. He does not let His people be hurled headlong.

When you hear His voice speaking truth to you again, you'll be refreshed at the change that alone will bring. You'll be reminded that He hasn't let go of you, and He never will. You're His precious child. There is no limit to His love for you. If He leaves you in your suffering, He's there to help you through it.

In His infinite love for each of His children, God stays away from popular, "new" religious fads. With Him there are no new gimmicks and no better ways. He only promises more of Himself and His ever-present help, more new discoveries in Him, and a deeper joy when we obey Him even in the hard times. When trouble hits, we need to give Him the chance to prove He can help us.

Actually, God works daily to prove Himself to His people. J. I. Packer, in his book *Knowing God*, discusses the adequacy of God as our sovereign benefactor. As an example, he points to the ways He proved Himself to Israel when He delivered them from slavery in Egypt and led them to the

Promised Land. He imagines God offering an explanation of His work on their behalf like this:

> "By saving you from Pharaoh and his hosts 'by a mighty hand and a stretched out arm,' by signs and wonders, by the Passover and the crossing of the Red Sea, I gave you a sample of what I can do for you, and showed you clearly enough that anywhere, at any time, against any foe, under any privation, whatsoever, I can protect you, provide for you, and give you all that makes up true life. You need no God but Me; therefore you are not to be betrayed into looking for any God but me, but you are to serve Me, and Me alone."[16]

Our God's abilities are infinite and His ways are past finding out. Our goal is to know and trust Him well enough to be positively certain of this. In Ephesians 3:20–21 Paul has a reminder for us.

> "Now to Him who is able to do immeasurably more than all we ask or imagine, according to His power that is at work within us, to Him be glory in the church and in Christ Jesus throughout all generations, for ever and ever! Amen."

---

16 J.I. Packer, *op. cit.*, page 243-244.

Epilogue

BETWEEN APRIL AND JULY OF 2004, God answered many agonizing prayers from the past for spiritual harmony and growth in my marriage. It took something drastic, and He did something drastic. As a couple, our walk in faith together deepened so much during that healing journey.

Matt began to truly lead me and our family spiritually. We all loved it then, and we still do now. After God rescued me from my fear boat excursion, Matt and I continued having spiritual conversations and sharing a genuine love for the Lord together. He's more devoted to praying for others in their health and life situations.

His heart is softer, and I can see the glory of my King in him. God enables us to share truth and be mutually encouraging. It's such a blessing every time it happens. When the Spirit leads Matt, or any of us, the obedience that follows is impressive.

Since her illness, Elizabeth and I have talked about one of my earliest questions before she became sick—"Is it worth it to me to suffer so a spiritual change of heart can take place in someone else?" We both agree. The answer is "yes!"

As we continued our conversation about suffering, I told Elizabeth how hard it was for me as a parent to watch my child suffer. I've always tried to prevent or minimize the pain of my children. Elizabeth gave me the following parenting advice:

"Let your kids suffer. They can learn the comfort of the Holy Spirit in no other way."

Through her illness and recovery, she got it. She'd seen her God at work. My wise daughter reminded me that parental efforts can get in God's way. As believers, we all need to be convinced of the value of suffering.

Our journey taught us that the Lord has actually designed and equipped us to live and prosper through trials and troubles, not vice versa. Scripture gives us a reminder.

"For man is born to trouble as surely as sparks fly upward" (Job 5:7).

We grow and mature in that process.

Jesus Himself experienced deep trials and troubles. He said we could be of good cheer because He'd overcome the world and its tribulations. He wants us to look forward to our future glory instead of looking at all that causes us pain in the present. He points this out in the following scripture.

> "I consider that our present sufferings are not worth comparing with the glory that will be revealed in us" (Romans 8:18).

Even though I don't eagerly rush to sign up for more intense suffering, I know one radical fact of the matter is clear—people need trouble. I think of a few Bible characters during trouble-free periods of time who could have said: "Ah, this is the life!" For starters, Adam and Eve had a perfect, beautiful home and the best relationship with God. They were deeply loved. All their needs were provided for and they had free choice. But they threw it all away when they sinned.

King Solomon also had an enormously blessed life. God gave Him more wisdom than anyone before or since, and he was incredibly wealthy. He had known the Lord and His blessing on his life. But he tossed it aside, as well, by turning to the false religion of his wives. Sin ruins the best of lives and opportunities. Our God, our healer, works non-stop to restore them.

As we came to the end of our journey, I saw many ways God changed my view on suffering. For one, He taught me a new prayer for those who are in deep troubles.

"Please work in the suffering, crisis, or trouble to fulfill Your purposes for allowing or creating it. Don't necessarily remove the trouble immediately. Use it to break, change, and heal lives spiritually. Finish the work You began."

The Lord taught me that is what matters most to Him—always.

Since this kind of suffering hadn't happened to me before, I remember wondering in the past how it felt when the bottom fell out of peoples' lives. It seemed so scary. Way back in the second or third week of the journey, the Lord gave me a glimpse of how it may feel. We'd begun to sense that some big things we'd relied on earlier may just disappear. For instance, Matt's military base could have possibly closed around that time, so he could have lost his job.

There had also been a crucial change in our family health insurance coverage and we had to drop Elizabeth from our policy when she turned twenty-two, four months before she became ill. She'd taken out a smaller policy through her school and we weren't sure if it would cover all her medical bills.

"What if we need to sell our house to pay these expenses?" we asked ourselves, bewildered.

We didn't know if that would be necessary, but we could have lost our house. When I thought of the former healthy life of my daughter, I wondered what kind of a future she'd have. I suddenly felt I was completely at the end of myself and my abilities.

When I thought about it, I realized all I really had for sure was the Lord. The times when I truly understood that fact were the times where real faith began for me on the journey. When I discovered He was all I could count on, it was very freeing. Life seemed so simple. I felt like a little child sitting safely on my Daddy's lap. He held onto me and I was secure. I knew I'd be okay.

In Elizabeth's case, after she got home from the hospital, we learned her policy only covered the first month of her hospital stay. That meant two-thirds of her care wasn't covered. The Lord moved and provided the means for paying the remaining huge financial need and we didn't have to sell our house after all.

Since her recovery, Elizabeth leads a healthy, active life. She worked full time with autistic children for three and a half years and she ministered to high school students in her church for almost five years. Today, she and John host an adult small group in their home and their family remains active in church. She has also hiked and backpacked in high altitudes. She loves going on trips, both short and long. She keeps up well as she meets the needs of her household.

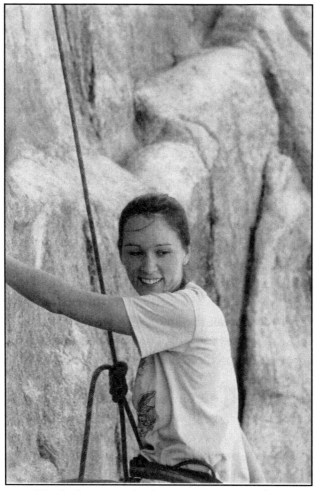

Elizabeth in rock climbing gear 1 ½ years after she got married

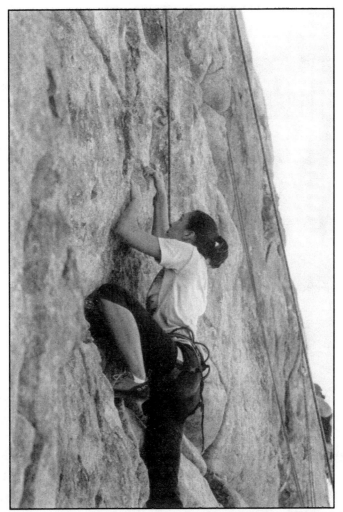

Elizabeth moving on with life

Nine months after leaving the hospital, she had a follow-up lung capacity test. She was told some moderate lung damage remained, but it was hard to determine the amount. Elizabeth left it at that. You'd never know she'd once been so sick unless she told you.

The most recent blessings the Lord has poured out on Elizabeth and John are the healthy births of their two sons, Levi Robert, in 2009 and Silas Matthew, in 2011. Joy abounds!

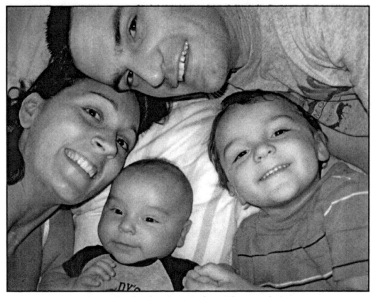

John, Elizabeth, their baby, Silas, and their
2 ½ year old son, Levi

We've all been the recipients of ineffective help that does a variety of frustrating things. It may make the problem worse, lead to more work, or make us feel terrible about needing help. Help that is unavailable when we need it is also ineffective. When helping efforts go awry, we quickly realize the person trying to help us doesn't accurately understand our problem or know how to help.

But our Ever-Present Help doesn't "help" that way. His excellent, God-sized help is totally effective. When He provides assistance, He has infinite power, skills, resources, and understanding. He's always available. His help perfectly fits the need, and even gets to the root of the problem. He exerts His helpful energy with love and compassion.

Together my entire family praises Him, our Ever-Present Help, for His magnificent assistance.

> "For I am the Lord, your God, who takes hold of your right hand and says to you, Do not fear; I will help you" (Isaiah 41:13).

Resources

1. Barlow Respiratory Hospital and Research Center, 2000 Stadium Way, Los Angeles, CA 90026, USA, (213) 250-4200, www.barlow2000.org.
2. Biola University, 13800 Biola Avenue, La Mirada, CA, USA, (562) 903-6000.
3. Passy-Muir, Inc., PMB 273, 4521 Campus Drive, Irvine, CA 92612, USA, (949) 833-talk, (800) 634-5397, website: Passy-Muir.com.
4. Cedars-Sinai Medical Center, 8700 Beverly Blvd., Los Angeles, CA 90048, phone: main switchboard (310) 4-CEDARS (423-3277), www.cedars-sinai.edu.
5. ARDS – Acute Respiratory Distress Syndrome, www.ards.org. Source of information and support for patients, survivors, families, friends, medical personnel and others affected by ARDS. This website takes you to the ARDS Support Center. Next go to Communications or Immediate Support, then click on Pen Pal Circle, and then go to Friends and Families that have a loved one in ARDS crisis. Find personal e-mail addresses included with contributed comments.

CPSIA information can be obtained at www.ICGtesting.com
Printed in the USA
LVOW100909110712

289613LV00001B/4/P